W9-AWY-752

SeXual Fitness

Hank C. K. Wuh, M.D.
MeiMei Fox

SeXual Fitness

7 Essential Elements to Optimizing Your Sensuality, Satisfaction, and Well-Being

G. P. Putnam's Sons
New York

Every effort has been made to ensure that the information contained in this book is complete and accurate. However, neither the publisher nor the author is engaged in rendering professional advice or services to the individual reader. The ideas, procedures, and suggestions contained in this book are not intended as a substitute for consulting with your physician. All matters regarding your health require medical supervision. Neither the author nor the publisher shall be liable or responsible for any loss, injury, or damage allegedly arising from any information or suggestion in this book.

The recipes contained in this book are to be followed exactly as written. Neither the publisher nor the author is responsible for your specific health or allergy needs that may require medical supervision, or for any adverse reactions to the recipes contained in this book.

Names and details of cases and characters have been changed to protect privacy and confidentiality.

G. P. Putnam's Sons
Publishers Since 1838
a member of
Penguin Putnam Inc.
375 Hudson Street
New York, NY 10014

Published simultaneously in Canada

Library of Congress Cataloging-in-Publication Data

Wuh, Hank C. K.
Sexual fitness : 7 essential elements to optimizing your sensuality, satisfaction, and well-being / Hank C. K. Wuh, MeiMei Fox.
p. cm.
Includes bibliographical references and index.
ISBN 0-399-14716-0
1. Sex instruction. 2. Sexual exercises. 3. Sexual excitement. 4. Physical fitness. 5. Diet. I. Fox, MeiMei. II. Title.
HQ31.W964 2001 00-057470
613.9'5—dc21

1 3 5 7 9 10 8 6 4 2

This book is printed on acid-free paper. ∞

BOOK DESIGN BY AMANDA DEWEY

We each dedicate this book to our parents,
for nurturing in us the capacity to love,
the curiosity to learn, the courage to believe,
and the humility to listen.

Acknowledgments

This book grew out of an immense need for people of all ages and backgrounds to realize that they can take control of their sexual health and wellness. Many generous individuals helped us along the way, allowing us to share our message of empowerment.

Special thanks to our literary agent, Janis Vallely, who saw at once the potential of the project and offered her patient guidance. Our deepest gratitude to Amy Hertz, executive editor at Riverhead, for believing in this important message and supporting us throughout the book's development and writing process. We owe our warmest appreciation to our editor at Putnam, Jennifer Repo, for her outstanding editorial work and constant attention to detail. We offer many thanks to Paula Page, our publicist, for her inspirational enthusiasm and spirit, and to Denny Kwock, for his wonderful friendship and constant resourcefulness.

We are grateful to Adria Popkin, who generously provided us with contacts in publishing, and to Nicole Wan, who selflessly shared her expertise and brought us to the people at Putnam. Many thanks to Stacy Elliott, M.D., a specialist in sexual medicine, for providing detailed medical information and the latest research as well as the case studies from her own practice. We owe tremendous gratitude to Aileen Trant, Ph.D., a nutritionist, for contributing to the meal plans and recipes, and for reviewing the manuscript. Alexandra Arch served very ably as a research assistant, working quickly yet accurately under tight deadlines. Our deepest gratitude to Carol Fox, who contributed recipes, ideas, and inspiration, and also offered detailed feedback on the manuscript. We would like to express our appreciation to Beverly Whipple, R.N., Ph.D. for her constant thoughtfulness and insightful comments on the manuscript. We offer a heartfelt thanks to David and Cecilia Lee for their inspiration and unwavering friendship, and to George and Jean Ariyoshi for their words of wisdom and genuine support. Many thanks to Jill Higgins and David Cole, who strongly endorsed this project.

We thank Jerome H. Kim, M.D., Mary Lake Polan, M.D., Ph.D., Diane Raleigh, Ph.D., Deb Levine, M.S., Linda Banner, Ph.D., Mitch Tepper, Ph.D., Wendy Leng, M.D., Thomas Ito, M.D., and Walter Chien, M.D., for taking the time to review the manuscript and offer their expert input. Thank you to Bill Lee and Kaye K. Kawahara, M.D., for your wonderful friendship. We are also indebted to all the Sexual Fitness Program participants, who shared their personal stories of success.

We owe our deepest gratitude to our families for their love and wisdom. Dr. Hank C. K. Wuh expresses his love and appreciation to his parents for their inspiration and support. MeiMei Fox expresses her tremendous appreciation to Carol and Galen Fox for emphasizing the value and joy of writing, to Dale Fox for his unwavering emotional and financial support, and to Jennifer Kramer for her constant encouragement.

Contents

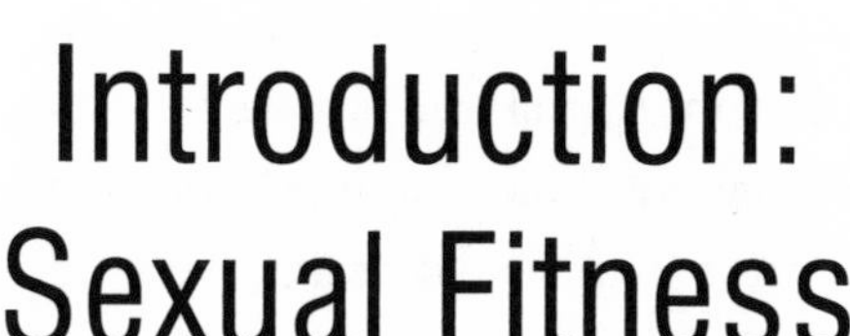

Introduction: Sexual Fitness

You can control your sexual pleasure and performance! Like most people, you may believe that you are trapped by your age, your genes, your general health, your hectic lifestyle, and other factors. But you're not. *Sexual Fitness* empowers you to make a difference!

Sex is one of the most significant biological functions in life. It is central to procreation, but it also plays a critical role in our enjoyment of sensual pleasure, our ability to experience intimacy and form bonding relationships, and our sense of self-esteem and overall well-being.

Yet despite the importance of sexuality in our lives, surprisingly few of us actually pay attention to optimizing our sexual health or "sexual fitness." And achieving sexual fitness isn't just about improving your sexuality. When you become sexually fit, you also become more physically and mentally fit. You'll enjoy greater vitality and better general health. The popular notion that, as we age, our bodies gradually deteriorate and our level of sexual enjoyment and overall health decline needs to be challenged. We can shape our own sexual and physical destinies. With the power of knowledge and the appropriate tools, you can improve not only your mental, physical, and cardiovascular fitness but your sexual fitness as well.

Sexual fitness is about understanding that it is absolutely possible for you to take control. Your sexual health, pleasure, and passion need not be left to dwindle over time. You can play an active role in maintaining or even improving them. When you believe in your ability to make yourself more sexually fit, you can follow the seven essential elements presented in the Sexual Fitness Program and achieve a more satisfying sex life in just thirty days! The program involves a combination of activities, which include enjoying the proper diet and nutritional supplements, controlling your intake of medications, stimulating your senses, exercising, getting good-quality sleep, and managing stress. These are habits that everyone can—and should—adopt. Whether you are in your twenties or your seventies, in basically good health or coping with illness and disability, the suggestions offered here will help you take charge of your sexual destiny.

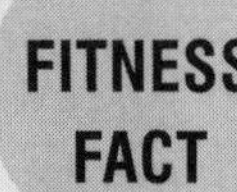

Adopting the healthy living habits presented in the Sexual Fitness Program may actually help you live up to ten years longer!

There are many advantages to sexual fitness in addition to better sex and enhanced intimacy. Being sexually fit will also contribute significantly to your overall wellness by motivating you to maintain a healthier lifestyle. A decline in sexual enjoyment and performance is one of your body's primary ways of alerting you that something may be wrong with your general health. So paying attention to your sexual fitness could actually improve your health or even save your life. And having safe sex with a dependable, trustworthy partner on a regular basis is, in and of itself, conducive to good health—it contributes to your psychological well-being, and can make you feel better and look younger!

While the Sexual Fitness Program suggests that you change some habits, the rewards make it worthwhile. You'll feel better, have more energy, and experience an overall rejuvenation. One part of this rejuvenation is increased sexual vitality and pleasure.

Sexual fitness isn't only about sex, though; it's also about intimacy and happiness. Some couples choose not to be sexual with each other and have adapted comfortably to this arrangement. Sexual contact—which does not necessarily mean sexual intercourse, but also includes all types of sexual activity—is clearly only one component of a loving relationship. However, for many people it is a critical one. Scientific research shows that marital satisfaction is correlated with sexual satisfaction. When either one or both members of a couple are sexually dissatisfied, relationships can suffer. Couples who choose to keep sex in their relationship and share a similar level of sexual satisfaction maintain an avenue of emotional intimacy and trust. Sexual fitness extends far beyond physical pleasure to your psychological and emotional well-being, as well as a sense of self-empowerment. It's a lifestyle decision—a decision about your overall health and wellness.

FITNESS FACT

Couples who engage in regular sexual activity rate themselves as happier than and are judged by others to look younger than their less sexually active peers.

The Sexual Fitness Philosophy

Sexual Fitness is based on a core philosophy that encompasses the following elements:

1. To value the importance of sexuality in our lives.
2. To pay equal attention to female and male sexual health.
3. To focus on prevention rather than treatment.
4. To integrate complementary and conventional medicine, but with emphasis on scientific validation through research and clinical trials.

What Sexual Fitness Means

Here are a few statements defining exactly what sexual fitness is:

1. *Sexual Fitness* is about optimizing sexual passion, pleasure, and performance on the physiological level.

In *Sexual Fitness*, we focus on practical and concrete steps you can take to ensure that your body is at its physiological peak. Part of this involves adopting a positive attitude toward your sexuality. *Sexual Fitness* concentrates on improving, through completely natural methods, the way your body functions.

2. *Sexual Fitness* is a natural, noninvasive approach to sexual health and wellness.

As complementary health care—the notion of preventing disease processes rather than simply treating symptoms—and the use of alternative medicine sweep the nation, people are seeking to maintain good health and avoid illnesses in the first place. Ongoing research suggests that we can enhance our general health by becoming physically fit: eating nutritious foods, taking supplements, avoiding substance abuse, exercising, getting plenty of sleep, and reducing stress.

3. *Sexual Fitness* is for healthy people as well as for those with sexual concerns.

Following the Sexual Fitness Program is like going to the gym—everyone goes to get more fit, whether they have a specific medical concern, are working toward a particular fitness goal, or simply want to look and feel better. When someone says "I'm going to the gym," it doesn't necessarily mean that he or she is out of shape. Similarly, you can have different reasons for becoming sexually fit, such as overcoming sexual dysfunction, enhancing your pleasure and desire, or simply getting in better shape overall. Achieving sexual fitness is not about meeting someone else's standards or expectations. It's a simple matter of setting your own goals and improving where you are relative to yourself.

Sexual Fitness is for you. It's for men and women of all ages, people who are healthy and those with sexual concerns. There are numerous reasons why you might be interested in this book: You may want to enhance the quality of your sexual experience; revitalize a flagging sexual relationship with your partner; overcome a specific sexual problem such as erectile dysfunction; or be empowered to lead a healthier, more vibrant life.

When you lead a busy, stressful life, as many of us do, it's common to feel that you have little time or energy for sex. When you are under pressure, your body goes into "fight or flight" mode, just as it would were you running from a tiger or jumping out of a plane. From an evolutionary standpoint, when your life is being threatened—when you are panicking and your body is telling itself just to survive—sex becomes the least important function on the priority list. So sex hormone levels drop, your blood vessels constrict, and interest in sex disappears. Because we have retained this basic evolutionary instinct, when life gets tough, sex is the first thing to go. When this is the case, as it often is, you need skills and knowledge to help get your body in optimal condition for sexual activity, so that you can make sex a priority again.

Alternatively, you may feel bored with your sex life. It's always the same old grind, and sex is not something that you look forward to anymore. You need motivation—specific goals to work toward that will improve your overall health and wellness, your outlook on life, as well as your interest in sex.

FITNESS FACT

There is no "normal" level of sexual activity. What is most important to sexual fitness is that you feel satisfied with your sexual drive, pleasure, and performance.

Another possibility is that you feel you could improve your sexual performance. Perhaps you have erectile difficulties, loss of libido, or other specific sexual issues that you'd like to overcome. If you feel this way, you're not alone. A surprising number of people—43 percent of women and 31 percent of men in the United States alone—experience some form of sexual dysfunction. You need strategies that can help your body, on a physiological level, to function better.

Whether you are in perfect condition or feel that your sex life could be much improved, *Sexual Fitness* can help. Your body needs certain nutrients, energy, and stimulation in order to perform well. An athlete wouldn't compete in a race without training, going on a diet specifically designed for peak performance, stretching, and preparing his or her body. So why do we expect that our bodies will always be perfectly tuned for sex? Instead, we might consider thinking about sex as if we were all "sexual athletes." Sexual athletes consume a diet that gives their bodies the nutrients they need, avoid smoking and other damaging habits, stimulate their senses, exercise, get plenty of rest, and take time out of their busy lives to relax. In other words, sexual athletes train to become sexually fit just as regular athletes train to become physically fit.

Many people assume that, over time, sex will become dull, their libidos will slowly drain away, and their bodies won't perform as well as they used to. They accept these events, along with wrinkles and gray hair, as facts of life. What they don't realize is that they have a choice. If they wish, they can take control of their sex lives. And so can you. *Sexual Fitness* explains how, by influencing your neurotransmitter and hormone levels and improving your cardiovascular as well as your overall health, you can put your body to work for you. Sexual vitality is within your reach. You can create your own reality—one in which sex drive, sensual pleasure, passion, and physiological function all remain at your maximum potential throughout your life. You can make it happen!

Are You Sexually Fit?

How do you know if you're sexually fit? Well, you can start by responding to this survey that allows you to quantify your sexual satisfaction. Please take the time to answer these questions when you are in a calm environment. To keep yourself honest, you should not allow anyone else to see your responses—this exercise is for your eyes only.

Although this tool offers only a simplified indication of your sexual satisfaction, it will provide you with a basis for measuring improvement. It should also give you the motivation to stick with the Sexual Fitness Program for the entire thirty days and beyond!

To complete the survey, read the question in the left-hand column labeled "Question." Choose a response from the column labeled "Rating System," then write the number you have selected in the column marked "Preprogram." Finally, add all the numbers together to

SEXUAL FITNESS SURVEY

QUESTION	RATING SYSTEM	PRE-PROGRAM	POST-PROGRAM
1. (ALL): Over the past four weeks, how would you rate your level of sexual desire?	1 = Very low/none at all 2 = Low 3 = Moderate 4 = High 5 = Very high		
2. (ALL): Over the past four weeks, how many times have you engaged in sexual activity, either alone or with a partner (with or without sexual intercourse)?	0 = Never 1 = One to two times 2 = Three to four times 3 = Five to six times 4 = Seven to ten times 5 = Eleven or more times		
3a. (MEN only): Over the past four weeks, how often were you able to maintain an erection adequate for sexual intercourse?	0 = Did not attempt intercourse 1 = Almost never/never 2 = A few times (much less than half) 3 = Sometimes (about half) 4 = Most times (much more than half) 5 = Almost always/always		
3b. (WOMEN only): Over the past four weeks, during sexual intercourse, how often did you feel adequately aroused?	0 = Did not attempt intercourse 1 = Almost never/never 2 = A few times (much less than half) 3 = Sometimes (about half) 4 = Most times (much more than half) 5 = Almost always/always		

QUESTION	RATING SYSTEM	PRE-PROGRAM	POST-PROGRAM
4. (ALL): Over the past four weeks, how often were sexual acts comfortable for you (e.g., no pain caused by intercourse or free from stress or anxiety)?	0 = Did not attempt intercourse 1 = Almost never/never 2 = A few times (much less than half) 3 = Sometimes (about half) 4 = Most times (much more than half) 5 = Almost always/always		
5. (ALL): Over the past four weeks, when you had sexual stimulation or intercourse, how often did you have an orgasm?	0 = Did not attempt intercourse 1 = Almost never/never 2 = A few times (much less than half) 3 = Sometimes (about half) 4 = Most times (much more than half) 5 = Almost always/always		
6. (ALL): Over the past four weeks, how satisfied have you been with your overall sex life?	1 = Very dissatisfied 2 = Moderately dissatisfied 3 = About equally satisfied and dissatisfied 4 = Moderately satisfied 5 = Very satisfied		
	TOTAL SCORE:		

calculate your total score. After you've completed the Sexual Fitness Program, you'll go back through the survey and complete it again.

Now take your total score and divide it by the number of questions in the survey, which is 6. This should give you an overall average score between 0 and 5, with 0 representing that you are very dissatisfied with your sex life and 5 representing that you are very satisfied. If you scored a 1 or less, you should consult a health-care professional for a detailed health evaluation. If you scored a 5, then you're just working to make your sex life even better. Whatever your score, there's always room for self-improvement!

The Seven Essential Elements of Sexual Fitness

The Sexual Fitness Program is based on what you put *into* your body and what you do *for* your body. Taking control of these seven basic aspects of your life will lead you to a new level of sexual fitness.

1. Diet

Consuming a balanced diet will give your body the raw materials it needs to function at its sexual peak. It will also improve your cardiovascular health and, therefore, optimize circulation, which is beneficial to erections and genital arousal.

2. Supplements

Key herbs and nutrients from natural supplements may help facilitate physiological processes involved in sexual function, boost energy levels, enhance circulation, and improve overall sexual enjoyment.

3. Medications

Certain prescription medications can interfere with sexual functioning, but there are specific strategies for coping with these side effects. Recreational drugs such as nicotine, alcohol, and caffeine must be consumed in moderation or they can seriously compromise your sexual fitness.

4. Sensual Stimulation

Stimulating your senses not only puts you in the mood psychologically but also has a proven impact on your physiology. Specially designed activities will help you to enjoy your sexuality more fully.

5. Exercise

Exercise improves cardiovascular health, boosts energy levels, reduces stress, and makes you feel good about yourself. All these factors work to enhance your sexual vitality.

6. Sleep

It's easy for us to cut back on sleep when we have a lot going on in our lives. But the truth is that getting an adequate amount of sound sleep is crucial to sexual fitness.

7. Stress Reduction

When we feel stressed, we often don't make time for sex. What's more, stress can shut off sexual pleasure and libido. Integrating basic stress-reduction methods into your daily routine can vastly improve your sex life.

The Sexual Fitness Program

In the last section of the book, you'll find a day-by-day program that will guide you to your optimum level of sexual fitness. It includes detailed recipes and three meal plans a day for the entire thirty days. You'll also discover creative exercises for sensual stimulation, stress management, and other fun activities, incorporating the seven key factors of sexual fitness—all designed to fit into your busy schedule.

The best part about the Sexual Fitness Program is that what's good for your sexual health is good for your overall health, as well. Many of the people who have followed the program report that they experience higher energy levels, feel more in control of their overall health and well-being, have more interest in and gain more pleasure from sex, and enjoy better relationships with their partners. So you can look at this book as a guide not only to optimizing your sexual fitness, but also to helping you lead a healthier, happier, and more vibrant life. And what better way to get motivated for a healthy lifestyle than knowing your sex life will improve!

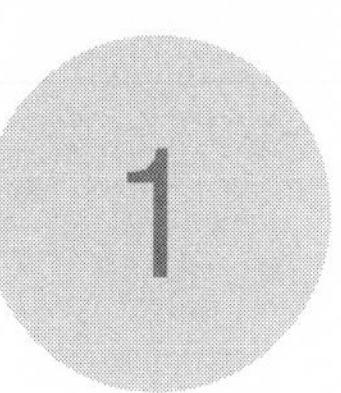

Diet

I begged Emilie to give me an oyster with her lips . . . I placed the shell on the edge of her lips, and after a good deal of laughing, she sucked in the oyster, which she held between her lips. I instantly recovered it by placing my lips on hers . . . —CASANOVA, *MEMOIRS*, VOLUME 6

Literary figures often compare great sex to food and great food to sex. Food can be suggestive, sensual, tantalizing, and arousing. People have used food to capture their lovers' hearts since the dawn of time. First dates, seduction, and romance frequently center on consuming a meal. Eating can be the prelude and the finale to lovemaking, and sometimes it's even the main course.

Food is, in fact, crucial to sexual passion, pleasure, and performance. From a scientific perspective, the aphorism "Food is love"—or at least "Food is sex"—holds true. Sexual fitness depends on a healthy diet. Only when your body has the raw materials that it needs from food can it produce the enzymes, hormones, and neurotransmitters required to make the entire sexual process flow properly.

During sex, your body draws heavily on many resources: sex hormones stimulate libido, circulation increases to generate erection and genital arousal, and neurotransmitters communicate all the messages zinging around your brain. Like musicians in a band, all of the systems involved—circulatory, muscular, hormonal, neural—must work in concert to achieve the desired result, a fast-paced song of emotions and sensations. In order to ensure that your body is well tuned and ready to perform at all times you must supply it with the nutrients it needs, the instruments that make up the band.

In broad terms, diet has an impact on sexual fitness in three ways:

1. Cardiovascular health: Your body requires adequate blood flow through the delicate vessels of the genital region for maximum pleasure and performance. Diet helps to keep your heart and arteries functioning properly.
2. Energy: In order for you to desire and enjoy sexual activity, you need energy. A diet high in fat and low in rich nutrients depletes your body of energy by slowing it down with junk that it can't use. A low-fat, well-balanced diet, on the other hand, can actually give you energy.
3. Nutritional building blocks: Your body needs specific amino acids, vitamins, and minerals in order to manufacture the hormones and neurotransmitters that allow you to have pleasurable sexual experiences. These nutrients, which come from the foods you eat and supplements you take, are the building blocks your body uses to generate the sexual response.

Give your body the great nutrition it deserves. When you respect its needs, it will respond by performing better. You are given only one body in your lifetime, so value it and treasure it as you would your finest possession. Even if you feel that you are currently in poor health, realize the potential you have to improve your state of wellness and don't give up. When it comes to taking care of yourself, there's no such thing as "too late" or "too soon."

Diet takes on particular importance as we age. As our bodies grow older, our metabolic rate naturally tends to slow, which means that our energy levels decline. We produce smaller quantities of sex hormones than we used to. A drop in hormone levels can result in a flagging sex drive, inhibited sexual response, or reduced sexual pleasure. In addition, our arteries often become clogged with cholesterol. Blocked arteries restrict blood flow, which can cause erectile dysfunction in men and decreased arousal and sensitivity in women. As a result, sexual performance and enjoyment may suffer. But they don't have to.

FITNESS FACT

Food is your body's fuel. By giving your body high-octane fuel, you can help it run like a race car.

Often, people dealing with sexual problems overlook the topic of nutrition. They are more likely to focus on specific health concerns, such as an enlarged prostate gland or menopause, and psychological issues or a relationship problem, than they are to include overall health and nutrition in the bigger picture. Yet stepping back and taking a look at your dietary habits can provide you with relevant cues you need to discover why sexual difficulties arise in the first place.

Take Jeremy and Susan, for example. These energetic, middle-aged best friends have been married for more than thirty years. They've raised children, changed careers, moved across the country—but through it all they've enjoyed a solid relationship and a healthy, active sex life. This does not mean that they make love every day or even every week, but they are accustomed to sharing the joys of sexual intimacy on a regular basis.

About a year ago, Jeremy started having trouble maintaining erections rigid enough to engage in sexual intercourse. He and Susan have a comfortable relationship, so they talked about the problem openly and tried to figure out what they should do about it. Jeremy considered taking Viagra, but he and Susan decided that they would prefer to try a more natural approach first.

When Jeremy spoke with us about his mild erectile dysfunction

(ED), we explained that his problem is quite common for a man in his mid-fifties. We urged him to visit his physician at once to determine whether his ED was a sign of cardiovascular problems or other health concerns, but reassured him that he should not be overly alarmed.

Then we asked some questions about his lifestyle. While Jeremy generally maintains his health by exercising regularly and keeping his weight within the recommended range for his height and age, his cholesterol levels are high. Cholesterol is the leading cause of erectile dysfunction among men over fifty, so arteriosclerosis may well have been playing a major role in his ED. We recommended some significant dietary changes to help him lower his cholesterol levels.

Jeremy loves ice cream. He has a bowl every night after dinner and sometimes sneaks one during the day as well, despite Susan's reminders about his cholesterol levels. We told him that he should substitute fruit sorbet or nonfat yogurt for this high-fat dessert, and that he also needed to cut back on his meat consumption—particularly hamburgers and steaks. We explained that by consuming a high-fiber diet rich in fresh fruits and vegetables, and cutting back on fatty foods, he might be able to reduce his cholesterol levels and improve his erections.

Jeremy agreed to give it a try. Six months later, his ED has improved. He still has some difficulty maintaining erections on occasion, but he and Susan are delighted to have the option of sharing the intimate pleasures of intercourse again. What's more, Jeremy is now highly motivated to eat well and exercise, maintaining his healthy new lifestyle.

Nutrition Fundamentals

In order to fully comprehend and embrace the dietary recommendations made in this book, it will help to begin with an introduction to the six basic types of nutrients—carbohydrates, fats, protein, vitamins, minerals, and water—and a new category of substances known as "non-nutrients." Once you are familiar with the terminology and the roles played by each type of nutrient in your body, we'll move on to specific applications to your sexual fitness lifestyle.

1) Carbohydrates

Carbohydrates provide the body with its main source of energy in the form of a fuel called glucose. Carbohydrates enter the body either as simple sugars or as complex starches. Excess carbohydrates are stored in the liver, muscles, and fat cells for future use.

Simple carbohydrates (those found in refined foods such as candy, cakes, ice cream, and other concentrated sugars) give you instant energy by causing your blood-sugar level to rise. However, a rapid drop in sugar and energy levels follows this burst, often leading to food cravings. Carbohydrates like these are also often lacking in essential vitamins, minerals, and fibers and are therefore referred to as "empty calories." They may temporarily fill you up and give you a brief burst of energy, but they do little to help your body function better for the long term. In fact, a high-sugar diet can contribute to obesity, heart disease, high blood pressure, and diabetes.

Complex carbohydrates (those found in unrefined grains and vegetables), on the other hand, take longer for your body's enzymes to break down into their simple sugars and glucose for absorption. They provide you with a slow, steady supply of fuel, leaving you feeling satisfied and energetic for an extended period of time. Most of the carbohydrates in your diet should therefore come from complex carbohydrates. Fiber, found in beans, grains, seeds, and most vegetables and fruits, helps satisfy your appetite because it's bulky food. It also improves intestinal health by giving your digestive muscles a good workout. Fiber plays a role in the management of obesity, colon cancer, high blood lipid levels, cardiovascular disease, and diabetes.

2) Fats

For many people, fat is what makes food taste good. However, fat is the most caloric, or "fattening" form of energy. Fat, also known by its chemical name lipid, is stored in the liver and muscles as glycogen but is most noticeable to the human eye as body fat, which can be stored in unlimited quantities under the skin. The body can manufacture most of the fat it needs but requires dietary fat to process fat-soluble vitamins (A, D, E, and K) and for essential fatty acids. Fat has other roles as well: It helps maintain healthy skin and hair, build cells, and insulate the delicate internal organs. However, it is easy to overeat fat—a problem that many of us have.

Cholesterol is a fat-like substance found in animal sources. Small amounts of cholesterol are necessary for producing sex hormones, among other tasks, but most Americans consume too much of it. There are two types of cholesterol: HDL (high-density lipoproteins), or "good" cholesterol, and LDL (low-density lipoproteins), or "bad" cholesterol. HDL cholesterol is associated with a decreased risk of heart attack and actually helps to remove cholesterol from artery walls. LDL cholesterol is associated with an increased risk of heart disease. It builds up along artery walls, causing a condition known as "arteriosclerosis," or hardening of the arteries.

Excessive fat and cholesterol consumption contributes to obesity, diabetes, cardiovascular disease, and many other health problems. But when you want to reduce the amount of fat in your diet, do not cut back blindly. Not all fats were created equal, and some varieties are less damaging to your health than others (see chart on the next page).

TYPES OF FATS

KIND OF FAT	WHAT IT DOES	FOODS THAT CONTAIN IT
Better Fats		
Polyunsaturated fat	Lowers "bad" cholesterol levels when substituted for saturated fats. Also may lower "good" cholesterol, however.	Canola, safflower, corn, sesame, and soybean oils; fish
Monounsaturated fat	Lowers "bad" cholesterol levels without lowering "good" cholesterol when substituted for saturated fats	Olive, canola, and peanut oils; olives; avocados; peanuts
Essential fatty acids	Linoleic, linolenic, and arachidonic acids (polyunsaturated fats) can't be formed in the body and must be absorbed from foods	Corn, cottonseed, safflower, sunflower, canola, and soybean oils; flaxseed oil; fish; nuts
Worse Fats		
Saturated fat	Linked with highest risk of heart disease. Raises cholesterol levels.	Animal and dairy products, processed and packaged foods, coconut and palm oils
Hydrogenated fat or trans fatty acids	Hydrogenation adds hydrogen to unsaturated fats, giving them more texture but also raising their cholesterol-making potential	Snack foods such as crackers, cookies, packaged baked goods, and candies
Cholesterol		
Cholesterol	LDL or "bad" cholesterol linked with increased risk of heart disease	Egg yolks, meats, oysters, shrimp

3) Protein

Protein, found in every human cell, is the most plentiful substance in the body after water. The body uses protein to create structures—from skin, bones, and muscles to internal organs and blood. This substance plays a critical role in maintaining health and wellness because enzymes that regulate chemical reactions, antibodies that help us fight disease, and hormones are all made of protein. Adequate protein absorption occurs only when you have sufficient fats and carbohydrates in your diet.

Twenty amino acids, which are metabolized from food or produced naturally in the liver, form the building blocks of thousands of different proteins. Essential amino acids receive that title because they cannot be manufactured in the body and therefore must be absorbed from food. This makes it critical that foods containing these nine essentials be part of your diet. Animal proteins including red meat, fish, eggs, dairy foods, and poultry are packed with essential amino acids. Vegetarian sources of protein include beans, grains, and some fruits.

4) Vitamins

Vitamins are essential for proper growth and development, the support of most bodily functions, and the prevention of disease. Vitamins are organic food substances found only in living things, meaning plants and animals. Many vitamins are required for chemical reactions that generate energy. The thirteen vitamins can be divided into two categories: water soluble and fat soluble. Water-soluble vitamins (B-complex and C) are not stored in your body and must, therefore, be regularly replenished through dietary consumption. Fat-soluble vitamins (A, D, E, and K) require small amounts of fat to be processed.

Scientists try to duplicate vitamins with synthetic substances, but the true sources may be better than supplements because of the special combinations provided naturally in foods. However, supplements can be helpful, particularly since much of our soil has been so depleted of vitamins and minerals due to overharvesting that many people argue that foods may not contain adequate levels of these substances anymore. Also, people with a poor diet—one low in fresh fruits and vegetables—should take supplements. In addition, the elderly often need supplements due to poorer digestion, absorption, and assimilation of food. Overconsumption of vitamins, on the other hand, can result in the loss of other nutrients and may interfere with normal physiological processes.

5) Minerals

Minerals, the same substances found in rocks, soil, and metals, are absorbed into the body from a variety of foods. They act as catalysts, stimulating chemical reactions and conducting nerve impulses. Minerals form the basis of bones, regulate blood pressure, and aid in the healing process. Besides these basic functions, minerals also help maintain the delicate water balance essential to mental and physical processing. Macrominerals, which are measured in milligrams, are needed in large amounts. These include calcium, chloride, magnesium, phosphorous, potassium, sodium, and sulfur. Trace minerals, such as iron, selenium, and zinc, are measured in micrograms and needed in smaller amounts.

Minerals cannot function without affecting other minerals. They also often require the presence of vitamins to work properly. For example, B-complex vitamins are only absorbed when combined with the mineral phosphorous. Meats, dairy products, fruit, vegetables, and grains are all good sources of minerals. Mineral deficiency results in illness. Consuming too much of a mineral, however, can interfere with the absorption of other minerals and nutrients, which may lead to adverse effects.

6) Water

Only oxygen is more essential to sustaining life than water. Circulation, respiration, digestion, metabolism, waste elimination, and temperature regulation all depend on water. Water dissolves and transports nutrients such as oxygen and minerals via the blood and other systems to the bodily organs. It also keeps the pressure, acidity, and composition of all chemical reactions that occur in the body in equilibrium. Aside from urination, water is also lost through sweating, breathing, crying, and evaporation.

We need lots of water in order to keep our whole body functioning well, and most of us do not consume enough of it. Dehydration can result in illness and even death. Most doctors currently recommend drinking at least 2 liters (68 ounces or about eight to nine eight-ounce glasses) of water or more a day. Don't consider sodas or juices, which are made mostly of water but are usually high in calories and sugar, as substitutes either. The pure, natural stuff is always best.

7) Non-Nutrients

Non-nutrients, which would be better named prenutrients, receive their title because they are not yet studied enough to be recognized as nutrients. Non-nutrients include antioxidants, phytochemicals, and phytoestrogens.

Antioxidants are non-nutrients that serve to remove harmful free radicals from the body. Free radicals are molecules generated during the metabolism of glucose and fatty acids and also result from pollutants such as ultraviolet radiation and alcohol. They attack cellular DNA, our genetic material, which can lead to aging, cancer, and heart disease. Antioxidants destroy and offset the damage done by free radicals. Vitamins A, C, and E and the mineral selenium are just a few of the antioxidants.

Phytochemicals are substances contained in fruits and vegetables that appear to have disease-fighting properties. Scientists are just beginning to study their effects on the human body, but preliminary research indicates that phytochemicals may help protect against certain types of cancer. Broccoli, carrots, tomatoes, garlic, and onions all contain these protective chemicals.

Phytoestrogens are phytochemicals found in certain plant foods, such as soybeans, that are converted to weak estrogens in the body. Phytoestrogens could play a role in the protection against certain types of cancer, such as breast, endometrial, or prostate cancers. The most likely risks of phytoestrogens deal with infertility and developmental problems, though very large amounts of dietary phytoestrogen would be needed for these risks.

Six Nutritional Steps to Better Sex

Now that we've reviewed the basic elements of nutrition, let's find out what your body needs and what it doesn't need in order to function

Guidelines for Healthy Eating

Recently, five leading health organizations joined to create one set of dietary guidelines based on the latest and best scientific research. The American Heart Association, American Cancer Society, American Dietetic Association, American Academy of Pediatrics, and National Institutes of Health all endorse this plan for healthy eating.

Four Basic Rules:

- Consume a variety of foods to ensure a well-balanced diet.
- Decrease your fat consumption.
- Increase your intake of fruits, vegetables, and whole grains.
- Don't overeat.

By the Numbers:

A person on a 2,000-calorie-a-day diet should get no more than:

- 10% of calories from saturated fat
- 30% of calories from total fat
- 300 mg of cholesterol per day
- 6 g of salt per day

at its sexual best. Let's also look closely to see how dietary habits have a direct impact on sexual fitness.

In general, anyone interested in long-term sexual wellness should consume a balanced diet. To help you get started we've outlined Six Nutritional Steps for Better Sex: Cut back the fat; reduce cholesterol; munch on more fruits and vegetables; eat whole grains, nuts, and seeds; add more soy to your diet; and spice up your life. We'll examine these suggestions so that you can understand how and why they have an impact on your sexual fitness and benefit your general health, as well as how to apply them when you shop, cook, and dine out. Following these basic steps will start you on the path to optimum sexual vitality.

1) Cut Back the Fat

There are many reasons why a high-fat diet is bad for you. First, a high-fat diet leads to heart disease and poor cardiovascular function. Clogged arteries prevent adequate blood flow from reaching the genital region, which interferes with sexual pleasure and ability to perform. A low-fat diet, on the other hand, can dramatically decrease cholesterol levels and even reverse the effects of arteriosclerosis. Whether you're twenty-five or sixty-five, physically fit or suffering from cardiovascular difficulties, consuming a diet that minimizes fat intake can help you ward off heart disease, feel healthy, and enhance your sexual fitness.

Also, consuming a fatty diet makes it more difficult to maintain a weight within the ideal range for your height and age, since all fats are high in calories. We'll examine weight issues further in chapter 5: *Exercise*, but realize that being significantly overweight can hinder your ability to enjoy a satisfying sex life.

The easiest way to cut fat is to reduce your intake of processed, prepackaged foods. Avoid fried foods. Slow down your visits to fast-food restaurants. When you do go, order salad with low-fat dressing instead of fries. Start eating more so-called "whole foods"—fresh fruits, vegetables, and grains. The next time you're in the grocery store, look for foods that exist in nature rather than those filled with chemicals

Know Your Fats

Bad Fats

- Butter, margarine, and shortening
- Whole dairy products: whole milk, cream, half-and-half, ice cream
- Regular-fat cheese
- Coconut and palm oils
- Mayonnaise
- Fatty cuts of meat, chicken and turkey with skin
- Fried foods
- Many packaged baked goods, candies, and crackers

Better Fats

- Fish: tuna, salmon, and mackerel
- Lean cuts of meat, especially white meat (turkey and chicken) without the skin
- Avocados
- Nuts: pecans, almonds, walnuts, peanuts, pine nuts, etc.
- Olive, canola, safflower, sesame, walnut, soybean, and flaxseed oils

and preservatives. Keep in mind that even the natural fat found in foods like avocados and nuts is better for you than the man-made fats contained in margarine, cookies, candies, crackers, and processed cheese.

2) Reduce Cholesterol

When patients complain of erectile dysfunction (ED), doctors predict that they are on the road to heart disease, or arteriosclerosis. Why? Because both problems arise when cholesterol blocks circulation in the small blood vessels of the body. Arteries become clogged with cholesterol the way the drain in your sink becomes clogged with debris. Just as water can't get through the drain, blood can't get through the narrow passageways of your arteries. This restriction is bad for your heart and other organs. It's also bad for your sex life because it prevents adequate blood flow from reaching the genital region during arousal.

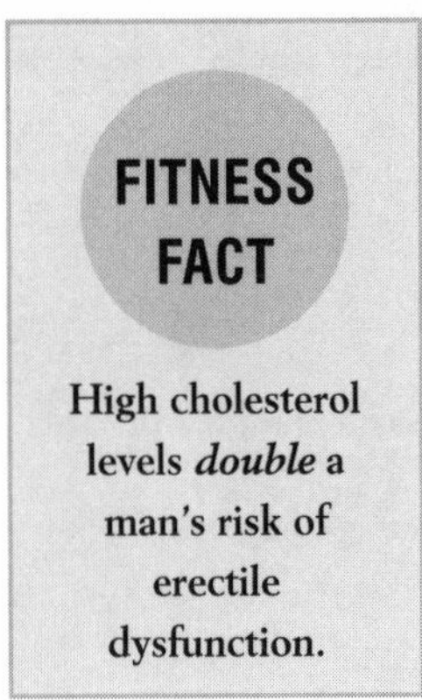

High cholesterol levels *double* a man's risk of erectile dysfunction.

While almost all the clinical studies connecting cholesterol to sexual dysfunction have been conducted on men, there is some evidence to suggest that the same correlation may hold true for women from the standpoint of circulation. Just as blood flows into the penis to cause an erection, blood flow into the vagina and clitoris results in lubrication and engorgement. With cholesterol blocking the arteries, this process may be inhibited. Women with arteriosclerosis may therefore experience a reduction in physiological arousal due to compromised circulation.

What can you do to keep your cholesterol levels down, and even lower your levels if they are already too high? Doctors often advise dietary changes. In general, you should cut back on consumption of foods high in saturated fat. Since cholesterol comes from animal sources, you can recognize and avoid it if you put your mind to it. Top cholesterol culprits include egg yolks (two to three eggs per week should be fine; try using more whites and fewer yolks), butter, cream, red meats (especially bacon and fatty cuts of beef and pork), oysters, shrimp, and palm or coconut oils. In addition, you can reduce your cholesterol levels by exercising regularly, not smoking, and losing weight if you are significantly overweight.

Sources of Cholesterol

- Egg yolks
- Whole-fat dairy products
- Fatty red meats
- Oysters
- Shrimp
- Palm and coconut oils

3) Munch on More Fruits and Vegetables

Fruits and vegetables provide you with many of the key nutrients discussed in the next section of this chapter. For instance, leafy green vegetables are excellent sources of folic acid, calcium, magnesium, and zinc. Fresh citrus fruits offer loads of vitamin C. Asparagus, long considered a sexual stimulant in cultures around the world due to its vague resemblance to the male phallus, is in fact a rich source of vitamin E, calcium, niacin, and other minerals. See the following chart to discover the sexual fitness benefits of many common fruits and vegetables that you can easily incorporate into your diet.

In addition to supplying nutrients for sexual fitness, a diet high in fresh fruits and vegetables is good for your overall health. Fruits and vegetables have been shown to lower cholesterol levels, which helps combat cardiovascular disease and improve blood flow to the genitals.

FRUITS AND VEGGIES FOR SEXUAL FITNESS		
FRUIT OR VEGETABLE	**KEY NUTRIENTS**	**SEXUAL HEALTH BENEFIT**
Apples	Magnesium	Fights PMS and menopausal symptoms
Apricots	Vitamin A Magnesium	Contributes to fertility Fights PMS and menopausal symptoms
Asparagus	Vitamin E Calcium Niacin	Contributes to fertility Fights PMS and menopausal symptoms Enhances sexual sensation
Avocados	Magnesium Niacin	Fights PMS and menopausal symptoms Enhances sexual sensation
Bananas	Vitamin B6	Fights PMS and menopausal symptoms
Broccoli	Vitamin A Vitamin C Vitamin B5 Niacin	Contributes to fertility Contributes to fertility Critical to sex hormone production Enhances sexual sensation
Cabbage	Vitamin B5	Critical to sex hormone production
Cantaloupe	Vitamin B6	Fights PMS and menopausal symptoms
Carrots	Vitamin A Vitamin B6	Contributes to fertility Fights PMS and menopausal symptoms
Cauliflower	Vitamin C Vitamin B5	Contributes to fertility Critical to sex hormone production
Citrus fruits: oranges, tangerines, grapefruit	Vitamin C	Contributes to fertility

continued

FRUIT OR VEGETABLE	KEY NUTRIENTS	SEXUAL HEALTH BENEFIT
Dark leafy greens: spinach, kale, chard, dandelion greens, collard greens, beet greens	Vitamins A,C,E Calcium Folate Magnesium Zinc	Contribute to fertility Fights PMS and menopausal symptoms Contributes to fertility Fights PMS and menopausal symptoms Contributes to fertility
Garlic	Selenium Zinc	Contributes to fertility Contributes to fertility
Peas	Vitamin E Niacin	Contributes to fertility Enhances sexual sensation
Peppers	Vitamin C	Contributes to fertility
Potatoes	Vitamin B5	Critical to sex hormone production
Strawberries	Vitamin C	Contributes to fertility
Squash: pumpkins, yellow squash, acorn squash	Vitamin A	Contributes to fertility
Tomatoes	Vitamins A,C	Contribute to fertility

When it comes to the glorious world of fruits and vegetables, you can't overdo it! Help yourself. Revel in all the wondrous taste sensations that nature has to offer. Here are some other tips for making the most of your produce:

- Eat fresh or frozen fruits and vegetables whenever possible. Avoid canned items, as frequently sodium is added and key nutrients are lost during the canning process.
- When possible, leave the skins on your produce rather than peeling (be sure to wash well). The outer layer is often the most nutritious and fiber-rich part of the plant.
- Get different fruits and vegetables every time you go to the market to make sure that you don't get bored with your diet. Don't be afraid to try something new!
- Store your produce in clear plastic containers toward the front of your refrigerator or in big bowls on your kitchen counter rather than hiding it away. That way, it will be readily accessible and attract your attention.

4) Eat Whole Grains, Nuts, and Seeds

A diet high in fiber and starch provides an important basis for cardiovascular health. Consumption of whole grains, nuts, and seeds will add both fiber and complex carbohydrates to your diet. This can reduce the risk of heart disease and contribute to improved sexual fitness.

Why are the health benefits of unprocessed or "whole" grains greater than the benefits of processed grains? Whole grains contain larger amounts of dietary fiber, vitamins, and minerals, which are frequently removed during processing. To add more whole grains to your diet, reduce your intake of refined pasta, cereal, flour, and bread products. Choose a whole-wheat bagel over a plain one, brown rice over white rice, and whole-wheat or multigrain bread over white bread. Have oatmeal or another whole-grain cereal for breakfast. Try to eat grains as they occur naturally—which usually means larger, chunkier, and harder to chew than refined grains. Even though they may seem unappealing at first, most people come to enjoy the flavor and sub-

GRAINS, SEEDS, AND NUTS FOR SEXUAL FITNESS

PRODUCT	KEY NUTRIENTS	SEXUAL HEALTH BENEFIT
Nuts: almonds, peanuts, cashews, walnuts, Brazil nuts, pecans	Vitamin E	Contributes to fertility
	Vitamin B5	Critical to sex hormone production
	Vitamin B6	Fights PMS and menopausal symptoms
	Calcium	Fights PMS and menopausal symptoms
	Folate	Contributes to fertility
	L-arginine	Necessary for erections
	Lecithin	Critical to sex hormone production
	Magnesium	Fights PMS and menopausal symptoms
	Niacin	Enhances sexual sensation
	Selenium	Contributes to fertility
	Thiamin	Boosts energy levels
	Zinc	Contributes to fertility
Seeds: flaxseed, sunflower seeds, poppy seeds, pumpkin seeds	Vitamin E	Contributes to fertility
	Vitamin B6	Fights PMS and menopausal symptoms
	L-arginine	Necessary for erections
	Lecithin	Critical to sex hormone production
	Magnesium	Fights PMS and menopausal symptoms
	Thiamin	Boosts energy levels
Whole Grains: oats, bran, wheat, rye, unrefined flour, barley, brown rice, cornmeal, buckwheat, spelt, sorghum, quinoa, kasha, wild rice	Vitamin E	Contributes to fertility
	Vitamin B5	Critical to sex hormone production
	Vitamin B6	Fights PMS and menopausal symptoms
	Folate	Contributes to fertility
	L-arginine	Necessary for erections
	Lecithin	Critical to sex hormone production
	Magnesium	Fights PMS and menopausal symptoms
	Niacin	Enhances sexual sensation
	Selenium	Contributes to fertility
	Thiamin	Boosts energy levels
	Zinc	Contributes to fertility

stance of whole grains over time. In addition, whole grains tend to be more filling, which can aid in weight management.

Nuts and seeds are critical to your nutritional program, as well. See the chart on page 31 for a list of the sexual benefits of grains, nuts, and seeds. Eat unsalted nuts and seeds with no added artificial flavor. You can eat them alone, or add them to salads, cereal, casseroles, and a variety of other dishes that you cook.

Ways to Enjoy Soy

- Soymilk: Plain, vanilla, chocolate, and other flavors available. Fortified soymilk has added vitamins and minerals. Can be used just like cow's milk. Drink plain, eat with cereal, make into hot chocolate, mix with tea or coffee, add to smoothies, substitute in recipes calling for milk.
- Tofu: Smooth and firm varieties available. Use smooth tofu for smoothies or "milk shakes," desserts, and recipes calling for cream. Firm tofu is best for stir-fry and as a meat substitute in many recipes.
- Tempeh: This firm, brown-variety soy is an excellent substitute for meat in most recipes. It's thicker and sticks together more than does tofu, and retains a meatlike quality when cooked.
- Soybeans: Called *edamame* in Japanese. Boil, salt, and eat plain by popping the seeds out of the skin and into your mouth. Often available preprepared in health food stores, either fresh or frozen. Also served as appetizers in Japanese restaurants.
- Soy nuts: Eat like regular nuts. Can be found in many health food stores.
- Soy-based products: Many grocery stores now carry products that substitute soy for meat, such as soy dogs, soy burgers, and even soy luncheon meats. Try these out and see which ones you like—some are delicious. Don't rely on these products for your entire soy intake, however, as they can be high in sodium and other additives.

PROTEIN FOR SEXUAL FITNESS

PRODUCT	KEY NUTRIENTS	SEXUAL HEALTH BENEFIT
Dairy: nonfat milk, yogurt, and cottage cheese; low-fat cheese; and ice milk	Vitamin A Vitamin B12 Calcium Magnesium Selenium	Contributes to fertility Contributes to fertility Fights PMS and menopausal symptoms Fights PMS and menopausal symptoms Contributes to fertility
Eggs	Vitamin A Vitamin B5 Vitamin B12 Selenium Zinc	Contributes to fertility Critical to sex hormone production Contributes to fertility Contributes to fertility Contributes to fertility
Meats: fish, shellfish, chicken, turkey, low-fat cuts of pork and beef	Vitamin A Vitamin B5 Vitamin B6 Vitamin B12 L-arginine Niacin Selenium Zinc	Contributes to fertility Critical to sex hormone production Fights PMS and menopausal symptoms Contributes to fertility Necessary for erections Enhances sexual sensation Contributes to fertility Contributes to fertility
Soy: soymilk, tofu, tempeh, soybeans, soy-based products	Vitamin B6 Calcium Folate Phytoestrogens Magnesium Thiamin	Fights PMS and menopausal symptoms Fights PMS and menopausal symptoms Contributes to fertility Fights PMS and menopausal symptoms Fights PMS and menopausal symptoms Boosts energy levels
Beans: black, red, kidney, lentils, lima, chick peas	Vitamin E Vitamin B6 Calcium Folate Niacin Thiamin Zinc	Contributes to fertility Fights PMS and menopausal symptoms Fights PMS and menopausal symptoms Contributes to fertility Enhances sexual sensation Boosts energy levels Contributes to fertility

5) Add More Soy to Your Diet

Protein plays an important role in sexual fitness since it provides many of the essential amino acids, vitamins, and minerals that contribute to enhanced sexual function. However, you should try to limit protein from high-fat sources like hamburgers, steaks, and sausages. Fish, lean white meats such as turkey and chicken served without the skin, lean red meats with all the fat trimmed, and plant sources of protein like tofu and beans are your best options. Most Americans get plenty of protein in their diets, so this should not be of particular concern to you unless you are a vegetarian.

Soy products are particularly healthy. They are low in fat and excellent sources of protein, fiber, as well as many vitamins and minerals. Consuming a diet high in soy and low in animal fat can also help reduce cholesterol levels. As we discussed earlier in the chapter, cholesterol is one of the biggest enemies of sexual fitness. Finally, the phytoestrogens in soy appear to combat symptoms of PMS and menopause, particularly hot flashes.

6) Spice Up Your Life

For thousands of years, people in various parts of the world have believed that eating spicy foods enhances the sexual response. In a way, they are right. Certain spices can contribute directly and indirectly to sexual pleasure and performance.

Chili peppers stimulate the nervous system, causing us to sweat, our faces to flush, and our heart rates to rise, simulating the effects of sexual arousal. This may explain why chili peppers are popularly thought to boost sex drive in many parts of the world. In Asia, ginger has long been considered a sexual stimulant and overall tonic for general health. Because it stimulates the metabolic system, ginger warms the body, which may explain why it is used as a sexual aid (its shape has also been considered phallic). Garlic may prevent and even reduce the buildup of fatty plaque in the arteries, thereby improving cardiovascular health. As we've discussed in previous sections, good circulation plays a key role in sexual fitness by ensuring that the sex organs are amply supplied with blood.

We recommend using plenty of spices in your cooking. Herbs and spices offer a very simple way to add variety as well as health benefits to your usual cuisine—with no added calories. They can also reduce your reliance on fatty additions to the meal, like heavy sauces containing butter and cream.

Key Nutrients for Sexual Fitness

Specific nutrients can have an impact on sexual fitness. These nutrients are the building blocks of neurotransmitters, sex hormones, and other substances in your body that make sex happen. Some of the nutrients highlighted in this section have a direct impact on sexual performance: They help enhance circulation or increase production of sex hormones. Others work indirectly by providing the body with more energy, which leads to increased interest in sex and stamina. When you ingest adequate amounts, these nutrients have the potential to offer an impressive boost to your sexual vitality.

A, C, and E Vitamins

Vitamins A, C, and E act as antioxidants. Antioxidants are crucial to sexual fitness, helping to protect sperm, as well as other cells and tissues, from damaging free radicals. A study conducted at the University of Chile found a correlation between low antioxidant levels and infertility in men.

VITAMIN A: Vitamin A is required for the formation of sex hormones. In men, it is also involved in sperm production and the maintenance of testicular tissue. Men suffering from sperm deficiency who take vitamin A with vitamin E may find that their sperm levels improve. In women, scientific evidence suggests that vitamin A is crucial to fertility. Vitamin A–deficient women have difficulty conceiving and carrying their pregnancies to term.

Dandelion greens, a tasty salad ingredient, as well as carrots, yams, pumpkins, eggs, meat, apricots, papayas, milk, broccoli, tomatoes, and green leafy vegetables are all excellent sources of carotene, which is converted to vitamin A by the body. Vitamin A can also be taken in supplement form.

VITAMIN C: Vitamin C is a powerful antioxidant. You can find this vitamin in citrus fruits, strawberries, spinach and other dark green vegetables, tomatoes, broccoli, cauliflower, and chili peppers. Some doctors claim that megadoses of vitamin C can cause the formation of kidney stones. Therefore, if you are taking large daily doses of vitamin C supplements, be sure to drink plenty of water as a precaution. Vitamin C is otherwise nontoxic.

VITAMIN E: You may hear vitamin E referred to as the "sex vitamin" because of the role it plays in the formation of sex hormones. People who suffer from vitamin E deficiency may have low sex drives. Vitamin E improves circulation by efficiently transporting oxygen, a critical factor in attaining peak sexual fitness since firm erections and female sexual response require adequate blood flow to the genital regions. In addition, supplementation with 600 mg of vitamin E a day has been shown to improve fertility in men who are subfertile.

Taking a supplement is recommended because it can be difficult to ingest sufficient amounts of vitamin E through diet—especially a low-fat diet—alone (vitamin E is particularly high in oils and other fatty substances). However, do not overdo your daily consumption, as vitamin E overdosing can raise blood pressure. Follow the Daily Value guidelines recommended by the U.S. Food and Drug Administration (FDA): 30 International Units (IU) of vitamin E a day. Vitamin E naturally occurs in beans, seeds, grains, nuts, eggs, fruit, and vegetables including spinach, asparagus, and peas. It is especially high in oils from vegetables, seeds, and nuts.

B-Vitamins: B-6 and B-12

B-complex vitamins are critical to the activity of hundreds of enzymes and to energy metabolism. They also play a role in the production of testosterone, the sex hormone that drives libido.

VITAMIN B-6: Due to its reputation for aiding symptoms of morning sickness, water retention, and PMS, women may want to take vitamin B-6 supplements. Vitamin B-6 is also crucial for men. A European study showed that low levels of vitamin B-6 are associated with peripheral vascular disease. In this disease, blood flow to the smallest arteries of the body, including those found in the genital region, is inhibited. Therefore, lack of vitamin B-6 may increase the risk of ED.

Vitamin B-6 can be found in yeast, bananas, carrots, cantaloupe, eggs, honey, oats, red meat, soybeans, sunflower seeds, walnuts, beans, and wheat germ. Do not take more than 200 mg of B-6 per day in supplement form. Doses above 2,000 mg a day can cause brain damage.

VITAMIN B-12: Supplementing the diet with vitamin B-12 may help overcome erectile dysfunction and infertility in patients suffering from B-12 deficiency. You can find this vitamin in meat, cheese, eggs, fish and shellfish, and milk. Vegans (people who eat no meat, eggs, dairy, or animal products) will therefore need to take a supplement. The Daily Value of vitamin B-12 is 6 mcg (micrograms) per day.

Calcium

Most of us already know that calcium builds stronger bones and therefore helps ward off osteoporosis. In addition, calcium fights symptoms of PMS. In a clinical trial, taking 1,200 mg of calcium daily for three months resulted in a 50 percent drop in women's depression, mood swings, headaches, irritability, and other symptoms associated with PMS. If PMS slows down your sex life, you might try taking calcium in supplement form.

In order for your body to properly absorb calcium, you must also be ingesting adequate levels of vitamin D. Calcium occurs naturally in dairy products, which are frequently fortified with vitamin D. You can also find high levels of calcium in almonds and Brazil nuts, green leafy vegetables, tofu, salmon, sardines, and seaweed.

Folate (Folic Acid)

Folate (also known as folic acid), a B vitamin, helps maintain general health and wellness. It appears to facilitate the production of dopamine, a neurotransmitter critical to sexual arousal and orgasm. When people lack adequate levels of dopamine, their sexual interest and pleasure both suffer severely. Folate is also involved in the development of mature sperm. Pregnant women are often advised to consume a folate-rich diet, as doing so may reduce the risk of birth defects.

The Daily Value of folate is 400 mcg, which can be taken as a supplement. Also, beans, grains, nuts, and dark leafy greens such as chard, kale, and spinach provide excellent sources of folic acid.

L-Arginine

L-arginine is an essential amino acid that facilitates blood flow to the erectile tissue of the penis by increasing nitric oxide levels. In addition, L-arginine appears to raise sperm counts and improve sperm motility (activity) in subfertile men. An article in the *Journal of Urology* argued that reasonable evidence exists for using L-arginine as a dietary supplement to improve male sexual function.

The particular foods highest in L-arginine include meat, nuts, seeds, and grains. Since L-arginine is an essential amino acid (meaning that your body cannot manufacture it), you must maintain a healthy supply of it by eating plenty of foods rich in the nutrient or by taking supplements. In order to increase the amount of L-arginine ingested relative to the other amino acids in food, it may be most effective to take a supplement.

Magnesium

Magnesium deficiency can cause PMS in otherwise healthy women with normal menstrual cycles. Therefore, supplementing the diet with magnesium may prove effective in combating symptoms associated with PMS, especially cramps. In a British trial, participants who took 200 mg of magnesium daily for two months noted significant improvement in symptoms of water retention, including weight gain, swollen limbs, and abdominal bloating.

Try taking 200-mg tablets of magnesium daily to treat PMS symptoms. Foods with high magnesium levels include apples, apricots, avocados, dairy products, fish, leafy green vegetables, tofu, seeds, nuts, and whole grains.

Niacin (Vitamin B-3)

Niacin helps to dilate blood vessels. It may be involved in triggering the so-called "sexual flush," the rush of blood to the skin of the face, neck, and chest that occurs upon sexual stimulation. Some people claim that by adding more niacin to your diet, you may be able to create a more intense sexual flush. They also assert that niacin supplements improve tactile sensation all over the body.

Niacin-rich foods include asparagus, fish, lean meats, grains, peas, beans, figs, avocados, dates, broccoli, and peanuts. If you take a supplement, be aware that niacin can cause stomach irritation and indigestion, particularly in people with stomach disorders such as ulcers or gastritis. Do not exceed the Daily Value of 20 mg without your doctor's supervision.

Pantothenic Acid (Vitamin B-5)

Pantothenic acid is crucial to the formation of sex hormones. In addition, this vitamin may help increase overall physical endurance. Postmenopausal women often lack pantothenic acid and may, therefore, want to take a supplement. The vitamin occurs naturally in beans, beef, broccoli, cabbage, cauliflower, eggs, grains, molasses, nuts, potatoes, and poultry.

Selenium

Selenium is an antioxidant essential to normal sperm development. Taking a selenium–vitamin E combination supplement may significantly improve fertility in subfertile men. In a Scottish study, men with low fertility who took a selenium supplement for three months had healthier sperm and were more likely to conceive than men in the control group.

Women require selenium when they are pregnant, breast-feeding, or lactating. Selenium deficiency can result in infertility, abortion, or retention of the placenta. At the same time, excessive amounts impair embryonic development, so be sure to consult your physician about selenium supplementation if you are planning to have a child.

Brazil nuts, brown rice and other whole grains, dairy products, meat, eggs, and garlic are good sources of selenium. However, selenium is often lacking in people's diets, so it is reasonable to take a supplement. The Daily Value is 70 mcg. Selenium can be toxic, but only if you far exceed the recommended dosage.

Thiamin (Vitamin B-1)

Thiamin has an indirect impact on sexual performance by converting carbohydrates into energy. People with low thiamin levels frequently suffer from depression. Thiamin uplifts the spirit and is, therefore, sometimes called the "morale" vitamin. You can acquire thiamin by taking supplements, or by eating the following foods: soybeans, beans, nuts, seeds, and whole grains. The Daily Value of Thiamin is 1.5 mg.

Zinc

Zinc is one of the most important minerals for male sexual function. It is involved in every step of male reproduction, from the manufacturing of testosterone to the production of healthy sperm. Semen contains high levels of zinc. Studies show that low levels of zinc can cause sexual dysfunction in men and may result in infertility; without enough zinc, the body becomes depleted of testosterone and sperm are not produced. Increased levels of zinc, on the other hand, help to extend the life span of ejaculated sperm.

> **FITNESS FACT**
>
> A half cup of raw oysters provides 750 percent of the Daily Value of zinc!

For women, zinc also plays an important role. Studies have shown that zinc levels drop during PMS, which leads scientists to believe that adding more zinc to the diet may relieve PMS symptoms. Adequate levels of zinc are also crucial during pregnancy, as zinc deficiency can lead to abortion, prolonged gestation, stillbirths, and low-birth-weight infants.

To get more zinc in your diet, you can either consume more fresh, zinc-rich foods, or you can take zinc supplements. If you choose to supplement your diet with zinc tablets, moderation is crucial: too

KEY NUTRIENTS—SUMMARY		
NUTRIENT	**DAILY VALUE**	**POTENTIAL SEXUAL FITNESS BENEFITS**
Vitamin A	5,000 IU	Crucial to formation of sex hormones and sperm
Vitamin C	60 mg	Protects sperm from free radicals
Vitamin E	30 IU	Crucial to formation of sex hormones and sperm
Vitamin B6	2 mg	Reduces symptoms of PMS, decreases risk of erectile dysfunction
Vitamin B12	6 mcg	Deficiency can cause impotence and infertility
Calcium	1000 mg	Builds strong bones, reduces symptoms of PMS
Folate	400 mcg	Facilitates production of dopamine, critical to development of sperm; helps prevent birth defects
L-arginine	*	Plays critical role in facilitating erections and vaginal lubrication
Magnesium	400 mg	Helps combat PMS
Niacin	20 mg	May enhance the sexual flush and tactile sensation
Pantothenic acid	10 mg	Crucial to formation of sex hormones, may increase endurance
Selenium	70 mcg	Deficiency can cause infertility in both sexes and miscarriage in pregnant women
Thiamin	1.5 mg	Boosts energy
Zinc	15 mg	Crucial to healthy sperm and testosterone production, prevents PMS symptoms, deficiency can cause miscarriage in pregnant women

* Daily Value not yet established.

much zinc interferes with the body's absorption of calcium and can actually harm the immune system. Be sure not to exceed the Daily Value of 15 mg on a regular basis. If you choose to get more zinc naturally through your diet, oysters, meat and fish, eggs, whole grains, nuts, pumpkin seeds, legumes, garlic, and spinach are all good dietary sources of the mineral.

The Sexual Fitness Shopping List

Fresh Foods

- Fruits: oranges, grapefruits, bananas, grapes, peaches, pineapples, apples, apricots, tomatoes, figs, and whatever else looks appealing
- Veggies: leafy greens like spinach, kale, collard greens, dandelion greens, and chard; broccoli, asparagus, artichokes, lettuce, cucumbers, and whatever else looks appealing
- Whole grains: brown rice, wild rice, whole-grain pasta, nine-grain bread, whole-wheat flour, oats, and barley
- Protein: tofu; fish; oysters; skinless chicken and turkey; extra-lean cuts of other meats for special occasions; nonfat dairy products such as cottage cheese, yogurt and milk; and beans

Herbs and Spices

- Cumin, curry, cayenne pepper, chili peppers; fresh herbs like basil, dill, oregano, rosemary, and parsley; garlic and ginger.

Prepackaged Foods

- Natural, low-fat packaged dinners
- Veggie burgers
- Soy products
- All-natural pasta sauces
- All-natural salad dressings and marinades
- All-natural, nonfat sorbets and fruit bars for dessert

One to Avoid: Tryptophan

Ever notice how, after Thanksgiving dinner, everyone seems ready for a nap? This is because both warm milk and turkey contain tryptophan, an amino acid. Although tryptophan is a precursor to serotonin, a neurotransmitter that produces a feeling of well-being, those good vibes do not lead to enhanced sexual performance—quite the opposite! Tryptophan actually induces drowsiness. So avoid substances containing tryptophan immediately prior to sexual activity in order to maintain high energy. In addition to milk and turkey, other foods with significant levels of tryptophan include cream and cheese, pork, veal, beef, halibut, and sockeye salmon.

Food for Sex

You may be in a bit of a panic right now. You might be thinking to yourself, "How do I use all this information about basic nutritional guidelines and specific nutrients? How do I put it all together?" Well, there's no need to worry.

At the end of the book, we provide you with meal plans for three meals a day, detailing what and how to eat in order to enhance your passion and prepare your body for peak sexual pleasure. The meals are based on the principles discussed throughout this chapter: They are low in fat and cholesterol; high in fiber, soy, fresh fruits, and vegetables; and contain the specific nutrients mentioned here. For most items listed in the menu plans, we include recipes. And just because these recipes are healthy doesn't mean they're not tasty! We've tried them ourselves, and we must say that you should not suffer on the Sexual Fitness Program. You even get to eat dessert every day.

Don't forget that you're eating well for better sex *and* for better

Hints for Healthy Eating

• Only keep food that you really need to eat in the house. Don't stock up on junk foods. That way, you'll have to leave the house to buy something if you're craving an unhealthy snack.

• Make fruits and veggies accessible and noticeable by keeping them in see-through containers at the front of your refrigerator rather than tucked away in a storage compartment.

• When you want to snack, reach for a fruit or veggie rather than crackers, cookies, cheese, meat, or something else caloric and fatty.

• Don't starve yourself. If you wait to eat until you're dying of hunger, you're more likely to cave in and eat the wrong thing—and too much of it.

• Eat slowly and talk more. Give yourself plenty of time to digest and fill up with smaller amounts of food. Your partner will enjoy the extra conversation and attention, as well.

• Eat more frequent, smaller meals. Eat when you're hungry, but only to the point where you're satisfied, not until you are stuffed. You'll probably end up eating more than three times a day but consuming fewer calories.

• Don't weigh yourself. Your goal here is to eat a well-balanced diet that will improve your sexual fitness and enhance your overall health and wellness. You may lose weight if you follow the Sexual Fitness Program, but stepping on the scale is often discouraging as you expect to begin seeing results more quickly than you do. Let your more comfortable clothing be your encouragement.

• Reward yourself—but not with food. Buy yourself a new outfit after a month of eating healthily. Or, better yet, treat yourself to a romantic and playful evening with your partner.

• If you cheat or fall off the wagon for a short time, hop back on. It's better to follow the program some of the time than none of the time. Don't beat yourself up over a small slip. Just go back to the program as soon as possible.

health. Eating better can potentially help boost your libido, aid your sexual performance, enhance your sexual pleasure, give you more energy, and result in improved overall wellness. The meal plans are about healthy living, and improved sexual fitness is just one of the many benefits that you should experience.

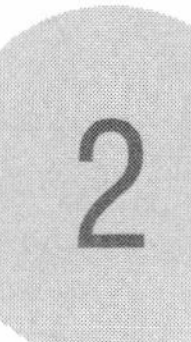

2

Supplements

Since the beginning of human civilization, people around the world have sought out magical foods and love potions to enhance their sexual abilities, passion, and pleasure. Three-thousand-year-old records from Babylon and China provide evidence that healers of these early cultures prescribed medicines made from plant and animal materials to help improve their patients' virility. The mighty Aztec ruler Montezuma, who believed that cocoa beans were an aphrodisiac, was said to have consumed fifty cups of hot chocolate to prepare himself for a night in his harem of six hundred women. The physician Hippocrates, working in ancient Greece around 400 B.C., prescribed honey for sexual vigor.

Some substances gained their reputations for being aphrodisiacs simply because of their physical appearance. The ancient "Law of Similarities" states that if an object looks like a certain sexual part of the male or female anatomy, then it must have an effect on sexual pleasure or performance. The rhinoceros horn, for example, resembles the male phallus and has been considered an aphrodisiac in parts of Asia for thousands of years. The ginseng root, a sexual tonic in traditional Chinese medicine, is said to look like various parts of the human anatomy: arms, legs, and even the penis. In fact, the Chinese name for ginseng, *ren shen*, means "human body." Today, scientific research provides us with evidence that quite a few of these ancient treatments—and some unexpected new discoveries—do indeed have these effects, due to a variety of physiological mechanisms.

Literally thousands of substances are, or at some point in human history have been, considered aphrodisiacs. The word *aphrodisiac* refers to a wide class of elements used to, depending on the interpretation and circumstances, rekindle lost love, make someone burn with passion, improve fertility, strengthen and lengthen erections, or even cause one person to instantly desire another. The dictionary defines *aphrodisiac* as a substance that excites sexual desire.

However, it is important to make a distinction between "aphrodisiacs" and those natural supplements that thorough scientific research has demonstrated have an ability to enhance sexual function on a physiological level. Substances do exist that have the potential to *gradually* improve your health and enhance your personal level of sexual interest and satisfaction. In order to avoid any confusion, then, we'll use the term *supplements* in place of *aphrodisiacs* when discussing natural products for sexual fitness. Supplements work to improve your body's sexual functioning by affecting neurotransmitters, hormone levels, and/or cardiovascular health. Over time, they may help you to achieve a greater level of sexual fulfillment.

The supplements reviewed here present several potential health benefits. Many of them have been successfully used for various sexual and nonsexual conditions for thousands of years by classically trained physicians and healers from cultures with a tradition of herbal medicine. In addition, these natural supplements generally have fewer side effects and cost less than do many over-the-counter drugs and prescription medications (see chapter 3: *Medications* for a detailed discussion of how drugs have an impact on sexual fitness). Finally, they often prove advantageous not just to your sexual health, but also to your general level of wellness.

At the same time, it is important to exercise caution when taking supplements. Many people assume that simply because these plant derivatives are natural, they are safe. In truth, botanical products can have powerful pharmacological effects. You need to be informed about their benefits, interactions with other medications you may be taking, and potential side effects.

Within the supplement arena, different opinions exist about which products work and which don't. Doctors in China and India have treated sexual dysfunction and enhanced libido through the use of certain plants, such as ginseng and ginkgo, for thousands of years, and continue to do so today. In Germany, some herbal remedies are more popular than pharmaceuticals. For instance, German women commonly use supplements derived from the black cohosh plant to treat menopausal symptoms, instead of taking synthetic hormones.

Over the past few years, natural supplements have gained widespread acceptance in America. More and more doctors and consumers are realizing the significant health benefits that can be achieved through the sensible use of herbs and nutritional supplements. What's more, researchers in the United States and around the world have begun to conduct scientific experiments to demonstrate that certain herbs are beneficial, and can possibly enhance sex drive and performance. At the same time, they're finding out which herbal treatments are no more than ancient myth and old wives' tales, void of real healing power. By preserving an open-minded attitude but also relying on scientific research, we can combine the best of both worlds—the alternative and the mainstream, the ancient and the modern—to find the solutions that contribute the most to our health and wellness.

Supplements for Sex

Below you will find a list of supplements that may make you feel more sexy, improve your circulation, or otherwise contribute to your sexual performance; ease PMS and menopause symptoms; help you relax and feel good; and assist with other sex-related health concerns. For each item, you will find a short description of what the natural supplement claims to do and how it works in your body, and scientific evidence for its effectiveness.

The items are grouped into three categories:

1. The "Yes" Category: Natural supplements that have a long history of medical use and have been well researched. Purported sexual benefits are backed up with scientific data. Clinical evidence shows that these supplements have the potential to yield noticeable results in many cases. Few of them have side effects when taken in the recommended doses.
2. The "Maybe" Category: Natural supplements that have, to support their effectiveness, hundreds of years of medical use, history, and anecdotes, but little reliable clinical research conducted on human subjects. These supplements may or may not hold up to further scientific examination. However, few of them have negative side effects when taken in the recommended doses.
3. The "No" Category: Natural supplements that have either been proven ineffective in the clinical setting or can be dangerous. These supplements should probably be avoided unless specifically recommended to you by a physician or qualified medical professional.

The "Yes" Category: What Works

To Improve Sexual Performance

GINKGO BILOBA Ginkgo is one of the oldest living species of trees. It has existed on this planet for the past 240 million years. In China and Japan, it is considered sacred and is planted on temple grounds. The leaves and nuts of the ginkgo tree have been used in traditional Chinese medicine for thousands of years to increase sexual energy, improve circulation, and treat respiratory ailments.

Ginkgo optimizes sexual pleasure and performance by relaxing muscles and increasing blood flow. Both of these activities occur naturally when the body is sexually aroused. Further stimulating these processes can therefore serve to enhance sexual fitness.

Ginkgo may prove particularly effective for people whose sexual difficulties can be traced to circulation problems since it helps the genitalia to become engorged with blood. One study, published in the *Journal of Urology,* showed that 50 percent of male subjects with erectile dysfunction (ED) who took 60 mg of ginkgo biloba extract a day regained their erections after six months.

Few studies have been conducted to test the effects of ginkgo on women. However, in a recent clinical trial, ginkgo proved extraordinarily effective for both male and female patients suffering from antidepressant-induced sexual dysfunction. A remarkable 91 percent of female subjects and 76 percent of male subjects experienced enhanced sexual response after taking ginkgo daily for four weeks.

Ginkgo works slowly, so plan to take it for at least eight weeks before you experience any effects. Ginkgo is nontoxic, but use it with caution if you're taking any blood-thinning herbs or medications, such as aspirin. Also, it may interfere with antidepressants that are monoamine oxidase inhibitors (MAOIs), such as Marplan, Nardil, Parnate, and Aurora.

You can purchase ginkgo in multiple forms. Please be cautious: Ginkgo is expensive, and many products offer minimal quantities of the active ingredients. Be sure to purchase only products labeled "standardized 24/6," which means that they contain adequate amounts of the active ingredients. The general recommended dose ranges from 50 to 100 mg a day. Avoid using unprocessed ginkgo leaves, including teas, as many people have allergies to them. These allergens are removed during processing.

GINSENG Ginseng is one of the oldest and most revered herbs in the world. Few people realize, however, that the term *ginseng* actually applies to three different plants: Chinese, Korean, or Asian ginseng (*Panax ginseng*); American ginseng (*Panax quinquefolius*); and Siberian ginseng (*E. senticosus*). We will discuss just the two Panax species, which are very similar. Siberian ginseng, a different but related species, is purported to improve endurance.

The gnarled mountain root of Asian ginseng has been central to traditional Chinese medicine for 5,000 years. The great philosopher Lao Tse praised ginseng's healing powers. The Chinese call it the "Cure-all" or "Elixir of Life." They believe that ginseng has a number of preventive and curative effects, including the following:

- Increases resistance to disease
- Stimulates sexual desire
- Improves brain functions
- Prevents headaches, fatigue, and exhaustion
- Restores "chi," or vital energy
- Stimulates circulation

American ginseng was used extensively by many Native American tribes for treating various ailments including cramps and menstrual problems, headaches, and asthma. Some used it in love potions. Tribal messengers frequently chewed on ginseng root while running between villages to help minimize their fatigue and boost endurance.

Ginseng appears to have a direct impact on male sexual fitness by increasing the production of nitric oxide throughout the body. Nitric oxide plays a crucial role in facilitating erections. Ginseng also increases overall stamina and vitality, giving users more energy. A study published in the *International Journal of Impotence Research* revealed that Asian ginseng effectively enhanced erectile function in men. Ginseng caused improvements in penile girth, libido, and sexual satisfaction. In another recent experiment, ginseng significantly increased sperm counts and testosterone levels in male patients with fertility problems.

Unfortunately, no published studies have been conducted to directly test the effects of ginseng on female sexual fitness. However, there is evidence to suggest that it may play a role in enhancing genital arousal in women. In addition, ginseng may offer another benefit to women: Research indicates that it may help prevent thinning of the vaginal walls during menopause.

American ginseng (*Panax quinquefolius*) and Asian ginseng (*Panax ginseng*) are both sold today in many forms. For example, you will probably be able to find ginseng teas, tinctures, powder, capsules, and even food products such as chips, sodas, and juices containing the herb. However, beware that foods fortified with ginseng often comprise only a tiny dose, probably not enough to have any real effect on your body. Also, the ginseng you purchase should contain at least 4 to

Ginseng Tea

Dissolve 3 small teaspoonfuls (3 to 4 g) of ginseng powder in a cup (approximately 200 ml or 7 oz) of boiling water. Stir and wait for about ten minutes. Strain the tea to remove excess powder. You may use the remaining powder two or three more times. The tea may be served with milk, sugar, honey, or juice. Take tea twice a day: once in the morning and once in the afternoon.

7 percent ginsenosides: You want to ensure that the manufacturers have a standardized process for including the active ingredient. Remember to purchase the *Panax* varieties. The general recommended dose ranges from 100 to 200 mg a day.

Both the World Health Organization and the German Commission E (a leading world source for information on herbal treatments) conclude that there are no known side effects to ginseng when taken in moderate doses of less than 300 mg per day. However, *Panax ginseng* may raise blood pressure in some individuals.

To Ease Menopause and PMS Symptoms

Premenstrual syndrome (PMS) is one of the most common health concerns for women today. For an estimated 30 to 40 percent of women, it has an impact on daily life a few days out of every month. Symptoms of PMS can be both psychological and physical in nature, affecting mood, energy levels, and sexual desire.

All women go through menopause as they mature. For many women, menopause is a welcome change, signaling the end of one period of life and a transition to the next. Some may find it a relief to escape from monthly periods, while others may feel saddened by the loss of fertility. For some women, menopause brings unpleasant side effects that may interfere with their sex lives. Symptoms can resemble those for PMS and might include insomnia, depression, mood swings, hot flashes, anxiety, low self-esteem, food cravings, headaches, breast tenderness, bloating, cramps, weight gain, fatigue, and decreased libido. Recent scientific research reveals that "male menopause"—health changes that occur as a result of a drop in hormone levels as men age—may exist as well.

While the natural remedies described in this section do not have a direct impact on sexual performance, they do appear to relieve menstrual and menopausal symptoms for some women. They are best used in combination with an overall health program, such as the one suggested in this book, which incorporates nutrition, exercise, and stress reduction along with supplements for optimum effect. Freeing oneself from the discomfort associated with PMS and menopause has the potential to enhance your ability and desire to have sex, and hence optimize your overall level of sexual fitness.

BLACK COHOSH Native Americans and, later, American colonists used the root of black cohosh (*Cimicifuga racemosa*), which grows in the forests of eastern North America, for the relief of menstrual cramps and menopausal symptoms. In Germany today, a drug made from black cohosh extract (Remifemin) is a popular substitute for hormone replacement therapy and is also used to combat PMS. Many clinical trials reveal that black cohosh is also an effective treatment for menopausal symptoms. In one study of over 800 women, black cohosh significantly alleviated menopause-induced irritability, anxiety, and depression. Other studies have demonstrated that black cohosh works to enhance vaginal lubrication and diminish hot flashes, headaches, and sleep disturbances. Scientists speculate that black cohosh works because it contains plant estrogen–like substances known as phytoestrogens, which seem to balance the hormonal changes that occur during PMS and menopause.

Black cohosh can cause some serious side effects at high doses (over 1,000 mg), such as dizziness, nausea, and headaches, so be sure to take only the recommended 40 mg per dose. Also, be patient because black cohosh takes a minimum of two weeks and up to eight weeks to build up in the body and create a noticeable effect. You should avoid black cohosh if you are already being treated for menopause symptoms with hormone replacement therapy or if you are pregnant. You may take tablets or drink it as a tea. To make tea, steep 1 tablespoon dried root in 3 cups boiling water for ten minutes.

CHASTEBERRY The chasteberry (*Vitex agnus-castus*) is the fruit of the chaste tree. You may also hear it referred to as "monk's pepper" because, in olden times, monks of southern Europe used it as a cooking spice.

Research indicates that the chasteberry is an effective natural treatment for PMS symptoms, particularly painful breasts. In a German study involving more than 1,500 women, 90 percent of the subjects found chasteberry extract helpful in relieving their sore breasts, bloating, and acne. Chasteberry may also be used to normalize irregular periods and treat symptoms of menopause. The chasteberry appears to balance hormone levels, but its pharmacological properties are not well understood at this time.

The generally recommended dose of chasteberry is just 30 to 40 mg a day. It may take several months to build up in your body and, therefore, for you to notice a change. It does not appear to have major side effects in most people. However, you should not take chasteberry if you are pregnant or taking hormone replacement therapy.

To Feel Good

CHOCOLATE Have you been looking for an excuse to eat more chocolate? Well, here it is. Chocolate—consumed in reasonable quantities—may help you relax and feel "in the mood." Montezuma, Aztec ruler and hot chocolate aficionado, was not the only one to believe in chocolate's ability to stimulate the libido. The notorious Marquis de Sade and womanizer Casanova also consumed chocolate, praising its wondrous sexual powers.

Chocolate does more than simply delight the tongue. It actually causes the mind to feel pleasure. Chocolate stimulates the release of endorphins in the brain. Endorphins are pleasure messengers that signal a feeling of well-being and happiness. Chocolate may therefore help you become more receptive to sexual activity. After all, these same endorphins generated by chocolate are released when you fall in love. In addition, chocolate contains L-arginine, a substance that facilitates erections in men and probably enhances genital arousal in women (see chapter 1: *Diet*). And a box of chocolates always makes a nice gift for your lover!

Supplements

KAVA KAVA Sexual pleasure requires a delicate balance of stimulation, in order to arouse, and relaxation, in order to enjoy. Kava kava is purported to create a calming effect without the side effects of a sedative. Captain James Cook, in the account of his voyage to the South Pacific in 1768, first described the ceremonial use of an intoxicating drink called Kava. The native people of nearly all the Pacific Islands have used the herb for hundreds of years in tribal rituals to create a meditative state and facilitate communication.

Kava relieves anxiety and produces a slightly euphoric state. It appears to calm the mind without interfering with proper functioning of the brain. Therefore, unlike tranquilizers or alcohol, kava leaves people with an alert mind and no unpleasant hangovers, and users do not develop tolerance. Also, kava promotes sociability, which can lead to an enhanced willingness to engage in sexual activities.

Most clinical research has focused on kava's efficacy in treating anxiety. One study found that kava induced changes in brain wave activity which were indicative of a sedative state. Several other trials have established that kava significantly reduces anxiety and enhances well-being, working just as effectively as pharmaceutical sedatives.

If performance anxiety or day-to-day stress plagues you during sexual encounters, you may want to consider taking kava to relax. The generally recommended dose is the equivalent of 60 to 200 mg of kavalactones (the active ingredient), usually contained in 3 to 6 standardized capsules, which can be taken in smaller quantities several times a day. You can purchase kava in capsule or tincture form at health food stores. You can also find a recipe for Kava Kava Cocoa in the recipe section of this book. At high doses (around 200 mg), kava acts as a sedative, and many people use it as a sleep aid. If you have too much of it, your legs may not allow you to stand up. Therefore, you should probably avoid large doses if you're interested in having sex later in the evening! Also, do not combine kava with alcohol or anti-anxiety, antidepressant, or cold medications.

For Other Sex-Related Health Concerns

CRANBERRY Many women are uncomfortably familiar with the symptoms of a urinary tract infection (UTI): pain during urination, the need to urinate frequently, cloudy urine, and even lower back pain. Men can also get these infections, but the rate of occurrence is far lower. Although UTIs are not always caused by sexual activity (physical activity such as cycling, and even panty hose, are other culprits), infection can arise after sexual intercourse, when bacteria can more easily enter and adhere to the genital and urinary tract areas.

Cranberry has gained enormous popularity in recent years as a natural treatment for UTIs. It works to ward off infection by preventing bacteria from adhering to the urinary tract lining. Scientific scrutiny reveals that it is highly effective. For example, a large study published in the *Journal of the American Medical Association* revealed that drinking 300 milliliters (approximately one 10-ounce glass) of cranberry juice per day significantly reduced urinary tract bacteria levels in older women after one to two months. Another study found that drinking cranberry juice for two months reduced the need for antibiotics among a group of women. This freedom from dependence on antibiotics is valuable, since the body can build up a resistance to antibiotics over time, making you more prone to other infections.

While the juice has typically been used in experiments, a recent clinical trial proved that cranberry supplements are effective, as well. Subjects who took 400-mg capsules of cranberry extract every day found that their rate of UTIs declined significantly over a three-month period. In fact, supplements may be preferable to juice. The high sugar content of juice can foster bacterial growth, counteracting some of the beneficial effects of cranberry. If you choose to drink juice, try the unsweetened or sugar substitute–sweetened varieties to avoid this problem.

If you frequently suffer from UTIs, consult your doctor about the possibility of using cranberry to prevent and/or treat the problem. You should drink 16 ounces of juice a day if you're symptomatic and 8 ounces a day for prevention—or take supplements. You may be able to lower the incidence and length of infection.

SAW PALMETTO More than half of all men over the age of fifty experience prostate enlargement, a condition known in the medical community as benign prostatic hypertrophy (BPH). When the prostate gland enlarges it can partially block the urethra, leading to symptoms such as increased urinary frequency and nighttime urination. This can prove very annoying and often painful. It can also interfere with your sex life.

Native Americans living in what is now Florida once consumed saw palmetto as a regular part of their diet. Early European explorers described eating the berry in the 1600s. The Egyptians used saw palmetto to treat urinary tract problems as early as the fifteenth century B.C.

Modern research tells us that consuming an extract of saw palmetto helps treat health problems related to an enlarged prostate gland. A prescription drug made from saw palmetto has been used to treat BPH in Europe for years. A review of clinical trials conducted during the past two decades, published in the *Journal of the American Medical Association,* concluded that saw palmetto worked better than a placebo to reduce urinary frequency and nighttime urination.

Saw palmetto naturally and effectively reduces prostate swelling without the side effects common to some prescription drug treatments for BPH, which can potentially decrease libido and inhibit erections in some men. Therefore, saw palmetto may be a less expensive alternative to drugs, and have less of an adverse impact on your sexual fitness.

If you believe that you suffer from an enlarged prostate, you should see a doctor before beginning any self-treatment. While BPH may be the problem, you need to rule out the possibility that your symptoms are being caused by a more serious condition such as prostate cancer. If you are diagnosed with BPH and your doctor approves, the generally recommended dose is 160 mg of saw palmetto twice a day. The herb may relieve symptoms of BPH while not actually reducing the size of the prostate, so you should continue to see your physician for this condition on a regular basis. Saw palmetto has been reported to be nontoxic and relatively safe even for extended use, but be patient—it may take two to three months to work.

The "Maybe" Category: What Might Work

The following is a list of natural supplements that have been used by people for hundreds and sometimes even thousands of years to enhance their sex lives or treat specific sexual conditions, but which may or may not work. At this time, the research simply does not provide conclusive evidence either supporting or refuting the claims made by many users and traditional medical practitioners.

To Improve Sexual Performance

AVENA SATIVA (A.K.A. GREEN OATS) Research indicates that *avena sativa*, an herbal extract made from green oats, may boost libido. Although the processes are unclear, *avena sativa* may work by freeing up testosterone. This sex hormone, which stimulates sex drive, becomes bound to a number of compounds within the body at an increasing rate as people age.

Male and female subjects in one experiment reported an increase in sexual desire and performance after taking an oat and nettle supplement. According to a *Men's Health* magazine survey, men taking 300 mg per day of green oats extract increased sexual activity by 54 percent. However, rigorous scientific research is still lacking, and we should therefore await further evidence of *avena sativa*'s efficacy before passing final judgment.

BEE PRODUCTS: BEE POLLEN, HONEY, AND ROYAL JELLY The legendary Greek physician Hippocrates prescribed honey to newlyweds to relieve anxiety and enhance sexual performance. Montezuma sweetened his hot cocoa with honey to keep his hundreds of concubines pleased. In fact, ancient cultures in the Middle East, India, and Europe considered honey an excellent aphrodisiac. After all, it is sweet and pleasing, just like sex.

The sugar contained in honey provides an easily absorbable source of energy, giving the user a so-called "sugar high." Honey is also packed with vitamins and minerals with known sexual benefits, such as calcium, zinc, and B-vitamins (see chapter 1: *Diet* for a list of these vitamins and minerals). Therefore, it is logical to assume that consuming honey may, over the long term, be of some small benefit to your general health and sexual wellness. However, there is no direct clinical evidence documenting honey's effects on libido or its ability to improve sexual fitness.

Bee pollen and royal jelly are both supposed sexual stimulants manufactured by bees and then processed into supplement form. Although it has enjoyed tremendous popularity in Asia for increasing sexual desire and potency, bee pollen has never been proven effective in scientific experiments. Also some people are allergic to it, so please be cautious should you choose to try it.

Many Asian cultures use royal jelly, an exotic substance that comes from the saliva of honeybees, to enhance virility. Anecdotal reports suggest that it might help alleviate erectile dysfunction and lack of desire, and may increase sperm production. Royal jelly contains numerous vitamins and minerals, but at this time there is little medical evidence to support its use as a sexual stimulant. As with other bee products, it is important to exercise caution when using royal jelly, as research indicates that it can lead to asthma attacks and severe allergic reactions. It's also very expensive as it is extremely difficult to obtain and preserve.

MUIRA PUAMA (A.K.A. MARAPUAMA) For hundreds of years, South American medicine men have used an extract from the muira puama shrub to cure erectile dysfunction and intensify sex drive. Its nickname is "potency wood." One consumer survey indicated that 51 percent of male subjects taking 1 to 1.5 g of muira puama daily reported better erections, and 62 percent claimed a boost in their libidos. However, the German Commission E, a leading world authority on herbal remedies, classifies muira puama as "unapproved" for sexual purposes due to a lack of scientific research. We'll have to await further clinical trials either verifying or refuting these results before we can move this supplement out of the "Maybe" category.

To Ease Menopause and PMS Symptoms

DONG QUAI The dong quai root is native to mountainous regions of China. It is mentioned in the first-century Chinese herbal guide, the *Shen Nong Ben Cao Jing,* as a treatment for vaginal infections, discharges, and infertility. In traditional Chinese medicine, doctors use dong quai as a general tonic for women and to enhance the female reproductive system. In fact, dong quai is often referred to as the "female ginseng."

Dong quai is an antispasmodic and may, therefore, be used in the treatment of menstrual cramps. According to a report published in the *American Journal of Chinese Medicine*, dong quai can tone the uterus, regulate hormone control, and stabilize the rhythm of the menstrual cycle.

However, scientific evidence regarding the effectiveness of dong quai for most menopausal and PMS symptoms is so far mixed. Many clinical studies demonstrating the benefits of the herb were conducted on dong quai decades ago in China. Also, in traditional Chinese medicine, dong quai is frequently prescribed in combination with other herbs. Therefore much of the Chinese research examines the effects of these herbal combinations rather than the effects of dong quai alone. One recent study of postmenopausal women conducted by Kaiser Permanente revealed no relief of menopausal symptoms with dong quai. It seems that the jury is still out on this traditional herbal cure until more research is done.

Pregnant women or those with endometriosis should avoid dong quai due to its stimulating effect on the uterus. Also, dong quai should never be taken with blood-thinning medications as it may thin the blood.

EVENING PRIMROSE The evening primrose (*Oenothera beinnis*), a yellow wildflower, grows along the East Coast of the United States. Native Americans have used the oil from its seeds for centuries to treat female health problems, as well as to heal wounds and treat asthma, the flu, and arthritis. Evening primrose oil (EPO) appears to work by regulating the body's hormone levels.

A review of several studies, published in the *Journal of Reproductive Medicine*, found that EPO significantly reduced depression, irritability, breast pain and tenderness, and water retention due to PMS. On the other hand, some clinical trials have found that EPO offers no help for women suffering from PMS and menopause.

We will have to await further scientific research before we have a clear picture of the effectiveness of EPO. For the moment, the evidence seems to weigh in favor of this supplement as a possible alternative treatment for some premenstrual symptoms.

To Feel Good

DAMIANA Used as an aphrodisiac by the ancient Aztecs, the damiana plant (*Turnera diffusa aphrodisiaca*) is native to Mexico and parts of South America. Its reputation as a sex aid may be due to the fact that the volatile oil contained in its leaves acts as a nerve stimulant, which can stimulate the urethra and cause the genitalia to tingle. Most people who take damiana do so because, they claim, it helps relieve anxiety and promote feelings of well-being. Damiana is also reported to improve circulation and balance hormones in menopausal women.

Unfortunately, at this time we have no hard clinical evidence either to confirm or deny damiana's efficacy. The German Commission E classifies damiana as "unapproved" due to this lack of conclusive research. At the same time, damiana is nontoxic and it may help you feel more receptive to sexual activity.

The "No" Category: What Does Not Work—and Might Be Dangerous

Next you will find a list of so-called "love potions" that you should avoid. In clinical trials, they have failed to regularly demonstrate significant benefit to the user. What's more, some of the substances may be dangerous to the environment or to your health.

To Improve Sexual Performance

ANIMAL PARTS Tiger penis, rhinoceros horn, bear testicles, deer antler, and other animal products have enjoyed a reputation as powerful sexual stimulants in countries across the globe for thousands of years. The apparent link between tiger penis or bear testicles and sexual potency is obvious, yet completely unfounded. While the testicles of male animals do contain testosterone, the hormones lose effectiveness quickly once the animal dies or the organ is removed. Moreover, these hormones are not present in the penis itself. As for deer antlers or rhino horn, these products are probably worthless: They're made up mostly of the same substance contained in human fingernails, keratin. Biting your nails doesn't do anything to help your sexual performance, either!

SPANISH FLY Although Spanish fly once enjoyed a reputation as an "aphrodisiac," it is actually a dangerous substance. According to legend, the Marquis de Sade spiked the drinks at a party with Spanish fly one night in an attempt to inspire an orgy—but ended up making his guests very ill instead! Made of beetle parts that are dried and ground to a powder, its active chemical, cantharidin, irritates the urogenital tract. The resulting itch and rush of blood to the genital area may stimulate erections and vaginal engorgement, making Spanish fly seem like a potent sexual aid. However, the substance can burn the mouth and throat; trigger urinary tract infections; cause severe abdominal pain, bleeding, and vomiting; and even lead to death. As a result, Spanish fly is now considered unsafe for human consumption.

YOHIMBE For centuries, natives of Africa and the West Indies have used yohimbe (*Pausinystalia yohimbe*), a substance that comes from the bark of the West African yohimbebe tree, to arouse their sex drives. It appears that the natural supplement yohimbe functions by stimulating the central and peripheral nervous systems. This may improve the transmission of sexual stimuli, thereby enhancing sexual feelings. In addition, yohimbe works directly to improve blood flow to the penis.

Despite these potential benefits, however, yohimbe has a long and serious list of side effects. Too much yohimbe can cause sweating, nausea, and sleeplessness. It can also increase anxiety levels, blood pressure, and heart rate. Use of yohimbe has been associated with seizures, kidney failure, and death. It can prove quite dangerous if taken without a doctor's close supervision.

A prescription medication made from the yohimbe tree called yohimbine, on the other hand, is accepted as a legitimate, and quite common, treatment for male sexual dysfunction. An analysis published in the *Journal of Urology* found yohimbine superior to placebos in treating mild to moderate, but not severe, ED. However, reported benefits have generally not been dramatic, and many people do not tolerate yohimbine well. If your doctor recommends treatment for

ED with yohimbine, ensure that he or she provides you with careful guidance and monitoring of side effects.

As with many other treatments for sexual dysfunction, yohimbine has been tested almost exclusively on men. One trial of the drug conducted on women with low sex drives concluded that yohimbine had no obvious effect on female sexual desire.

The Sexual Fitness Nutritional Supplement Program

Like chapter 1: *Diet*, this chapter contains a great deal of information about how much of which substances to consume when and for what reasons. You may be feeling overwhelmed with advice and alternatives. In order to help start you on the path to optimum sexual fitness, the next part of the chapter provides you with a recommended daily supplement program. This supplement program combines carefully selected ingredients from chapters 1 and 2 into daily formulations for male and female sexual fitness based on clinical research reports. By following the Sexual Fitness Supplement Program, you'll know how much of each substance to take and in what combination.

Taking supplements may ensure that you get the amount of key nutrients you need to reach your full sexual potential. However, it is also possible to get the vitamins and minerals you need for peak sexual fitness from a well-balanced diet. In this case, you need take only the recommended herbs.

The Sexual Fitness Supplement Program combines minerals, vitamins, and herbs into a formula designed for sexual vitality, pleasure, and performance. In traditional Chinese medicine, herbs are usually combined rather than taken alone. The effects of one ingredient can sometimes enhance the effects of another. It is the synergy of elements that has the most impact.

RECOMMENDED SUPPLEMENT PROGRAM FOR MALE SEXUAL FITNESS		
SUBSTANCE	DAILY DOSE	EFFECT
American ginseng	100 mg	Boosts overall energy levels
Korean ginseng	100 mg	Increases sex drive, sperm count, and overall vitality
Ginkgo biloba	50 mg	Improves blood flow to the penis; boosts energy
L-arginine	3,000 mg	Facilitates erections and genital arousal; raises sperm count and motility (activity)
Vitamin A	5,000 IU	Involved in sperm production; crucial to formation of sex hormones
Vitamin C	60 mg	Helps protect sperm from harmful toxins
Vitamin E	30 IU	Needed to form sex hormones; improves circulation
Vitamin B-5 (pantothenic acid)	10 mg	Crucial to formation of sex hormones; increases physical endurance
Vitamin B-6	2 mg	Enhances peripheral blood flow
Vitamin B-12	6 mcg	Insufficient amounts may contribute to impotence and infertility
Folate (folic acid)	400 mcg	Crucial to development of sperm
Niacin	20 mg	May enhance sexual flush
Selenium	20 mg	Essential to sperm development
Thiamin	1.5 mg	Increases overall energy levels
Zinc	15 mg	Required for production of sex hormones and healthy sperm

RECOMMENDED SUPPLEMENT PROGRAM FOR FEMALE SEXUAL FITNESS

SUBSTANCE	DAILY DOSE	EFFECT
Korean ginseng	100 mg	Increases overall vitality
Ginkgo biloba	50 mg	Improves blood flow to the genital region; boosts energy levels
L-arginine	2500 mg	May facilitate circulation to genitalia
Damiana	50 mg	Reduces anxiety; may be sexual stimulant
Vitamin A	5000 IU	Crucial to formation of sex hormones; contributes to ovarian fertility
Vitamin C	60 mg	Helps protect reproductive organs from harmful toxins
Vitamin E	30 IU	Needed to form sex hormones; improves circulation; compensates for low estrogen levels
Vitamin B-5 (pantothenic acid)	10 mg	Crucial to formation of sex hormones; increases physical endurance
Vitamin B-6	2 mg	Eases symptoms of PMS and menopause; enhances peripheral blood flow
Vitamin B-12	6 mcg	Low levels may contribute to infertility
Iron	9 mg	Often deficient in women; needed for blood to carry adequate amounts of oxygen
Folate (folic acid)	400 mcg	Helps prevent birth defects when taken during pregnancy
Niacin	20 mg	May enhance sexual flush

continued

SUBSTANCE	DAILY DOSE	EFFECT
Riboflavin	1.7 mg	Helpful to combat stress and fatigue
Biotin	300 mcg	Involved in metabolic processes to convert fat and carbohydrates into energy
Thiamin	1.5 mg	Increases overall energy levels
Zinc	7.5 mg	Crucial for vaginal lubrication; reduces PMS symptoms
Calcium	500 mg	Reduces symptoms of PMS; protects against osteoporosis

In a double-blind, placebo-controlled study, men with mild to severe erectile dysfunction followed the Sexual Fitness Supplement Program for four weeks. Over 80 percent reported improvements in ability to maintain an erection during intercourse and overall satisfaction with their sex lives, with few to no side effects.

David was one of the study participants. He is a sixty-year-old general manager of an export firm. He had difficulty sustaining an erection during intercourse until he followed the Sexual Fitness Supplement Program. After one month, David reported, "The effect of [the supplement program] is immediate and unmistakable. It brings a sexual readiness and capacity that has to be felt to be believed. Also its effect on my overall circulation system is extremely gratifying . . . My sexual balance is restored. And it doesn't cause an uncomfortable flushing sensation like the medicine I have tried does. Its effect on my sexual confidence is deeply satisfying."

David has continued to take the supplements ever since. He says that he loves the way they work with his body.

Women who were moderately to significantly dissatisfied with their sex lives volunteered to participate in the double-blind, placebo-controlled study of the female Sexual Fitness Supplement Program. After four weeks, over 70 percent of participants reported enhanced sexual desire and greater satisfaction with their overall sex lives. In addition, a significant number of women experienced improved clitoral sensation, a reduction of vaginal dryness, and increased frequency of intercourse.

Diane is one woman who feels she has benefited from following the Sexual Fitness Supplement Program. She was forty-nine years old when she went looking for advice about how to improve her sex drive. She ate a healthy diet and maintained an active lifestyle. Every morning, she would wake up before dawn and go for a ride on her horse. In recent years, however, Diane felt more and more tired in the mornings. She noticed a simultaneous decline in her libido.

Within a few weeks of starting the supplement program, Diane said, she noticed a skip in her step. She "felt healthier and more alert." She began waking up before her alarm even sounded and would take longer horseback rides. When she talked about improvements to her sex life, she turned red. "I haven't been this way since I was a teenager!" she exclaimed. Diane now takes the supplements every morning without fail. "I love my supplements. I won't go without them," she declares emphatically.

Unfortunately, you can't trust all supplements from all manufacturers. While some supplements can effectively contribute to your sex life, none of them can provide an instant erection, surefire seduction method, or overnight passion producer. With unreliable sources of nutritional supplements out there, you need to know which products you can trust. Here are some tips to help you purchase only supplements of the highest quality:

1. Look for extensive information on or in the product packaging. The ingredients and recommended dosage should be clearly displayed.

2. Buy only products that say they use "standardized" quantities. This implies that the manufacturers have included an effective and reliable percentage of the active ingredients.

3. Check for scientific research. The best products will have data and reports to back up their effectiveness. Look for information about clinical studies and, if it's available, ask for a copy of the results. Valid research should be published in a medical journal, and should be placebo controlled in design.

4. Purchase your supplements from a reputable source, such as a respected health food store or pharmacy. Carefully investigate all Web sites selling natural supplements to make sure the company is reputable.

5. Ask questions. If you are not certain about the quality or effectiveness of a product, look at the company's Web site for information, call the customer service line, or contact the company in some way to ask your questions.

6. Talk to your doctor. Remember to always ask your physician before beginning any new natural supplement or dietary regimen. Bring the product in with you to your appointment so that your doctor can take a look at the information.

7. Listen to your body. After taking supplements for the suggested amount of time, you should notice a change in how you feel. If not, be sure to reevaluate.

Optimizing your sexual fitness should also improve your overall health. Remember that what is good for your sexual pleasure and performance is good for your body, and what's good for your body will contribute to your general well-being. The supplements recommended here not only contribute to enhanced libido and arousal, performance, and pleasure but also potentially increase vigor, improve circulation, reduce stress, and even help fight illness. Following the Sexual Fitness Program will mean that you are adopting healthy habits for life.

Consuming a nutritious, well-balanced diet and taking supplements are the first steps on this path.

Nevertheless, supplements are not necessarily the answer for every person or every problem. If you suffer from sexual dysfunction, you should definitely consult your physician in order to determine the root cause of the problem and treat it appropriately. Often, sexual difficulties are a sign of a more serious, underlying illness or condition such as heart disease or diabetes. Be sure that you understand what is going on with your body, and how taking supplements might influence you.

Here are some commonsense cautions to help you figure out what to take and when. They apply not just to the Sexual Fitness Nutritional Supplement Program, but to any herbal or nutritional supplement plan that you would like to try:

1. Do not begin taking any supplement without first consulting your doctor. Many people assume that since herbs are natural, they must be safe. However, a supplement may react with a specific health condition or medication that you are taking.
2. Follow instructions. Many people may think, "If a little is good, more must be better!" However, in most cases this belief simply does not hold true. Always take the exact dosage recommended on the bottle or follow your doctor's instructions. Remember that most herbs require consistent use for an extended period of time to build up in your system and take effect. Look for slow, steady improvement—not instant change. Don't overdo it. Otherwise you may be putting yourself at serious risk for side effects.
3. You should probably avoid herbs altogether if you are pregnant, nursing, or lactating. We simply do not have enough long-term research to know what is safe for pregnant women and the life developing inside them. Play it safe. On the other hand, many herbs are purported to enhance fertility, so if you are trying to conceive you might want to consider a supplement program. Again, consult with your physician under all circumstances.

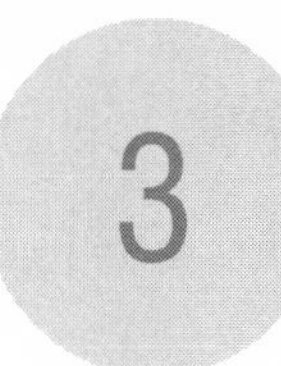

3

Medications

Matthew is in his early sixties and retired. He enjoyed a stable sex life with only occasional erectile difficulties until two years ago, when he started taking antihypertensives. While his blood pressure improved as a result of the medication, he also noticed an unwanted side effect—a significant decline in his ability to sustain an erection during intercourse. His doctor explained that this was a common problem for people on antihypertensives and suggested Viagra for Matthew's erectile issues. But Matthew did not want to take medication for his sex life. He decided to try the Sexual Fitness Program instead.

Matthew improved his eating habits and started exercising. As a result, he's been feeling better about himself and has more energy. His doctor has even been able to reduce Matthew's antihypertensive medication dose. Six months later Matthew reports, "My desire has improved. I'm having sex more often. I'm able to have sex with my wife, and sometimes I can even have an orgasm during intercourse. A month ago, we made love twice in a twenty-four-hour period. I haven't been able to do that in umpteen years. The results have been very consistent since I began [the program]. My desire and ability have done nothing but go up."

Matthew's antihypertensives represent just one class of drugs with negative sexual side effects. Several common prescription medications and many recreational drugs can inhibit libido, sexual response, and pleasure. Some pro-sexual chemicals also exist, but for the most part, drugs have the potential to detract from your sexual fitness. Fortunately, you can make a difference.

Sexual fitness, like most physical processes, depends on input and output. "Input" refers to what you take into your body, whereas "output" is the term for what you do with your body. "Input" comprises more than just what you eat. It encompasses everything that you consume, from sandwiches and vitamin tablets to coffee, alcohol and prescription medications. You can strive to be free from as many substances as possible, minimizing your input of damaging products. You can also optimize your sexual fitness while on substances that you are required to take for medical purposes.

The first step toward enhanced sexual pleasure, passion, and performance lies in understanding the potential side effects of drugs that you're taking. Many of us take prescription medications. Once you become aware of the issues surrounding your particular drug regimen, you can talk with your doctor about strategies for dealing with them. What's more, when you engage in the Sexual Fitness Program, like Matthew you may find that you have less need of certain medications.

Remember that you have the ability to make your sex life more satisfying than ever. Get started today!

Medications

Many of us take prescription or over-the-counter (OTC) medications on a regular basis. Yet few of us probably realize the impact they can have on our sex lives. Drugs can limit blood flow to the genital region, cause vaginal dryness, decrease libido, and alter levels of key neurotransmitters and hormones involved in sexual function. Common culprits include antihypertensives, anti-ulcer drugs, antidepressants, and even antihistamines that you might take for colds or allergies. For example, an ulcer treatment called Cimetidine decreases testosterone levels, which can lead to a reduction in sexual interest.

FITNESS FACT

About one in four cases of erectile dysfunction are caused by medications.

Sarah is a generally healthy woman whose sex drive was affected by prescription medication. She received a diagnosis of clinical depression shortly before her fortieth birthday. After years of struggling with what she believed to be an early midlife crisis, she was told by doctors that she actually suffered from a chemical imbalance in her brain. Relieved to discover that she was not completely to blame for her moodiness, Sarah began taking antidepressants. Within a week, she felt better, as if a tremendous load had been lifted.

Months later, however, Sarah realized that she was experiencing another problem. Although her dark moods had been alleviated, she no longer had any desire to engage in sexual activity. When she did have sex, she was rarely able to achieve orgasm.

Sarah asked her doctor about this unexpected change. He told her that many antidepressants cause a drop in libido. He switched her to a different antidepressant known for its lack of sexual side effects. With this new medication, Sarah happily discovered that her libido returned.

It is not within the scope of this book to review the sexual side effects of every medication. However, you will find an overview of the most common drugs that interfere with sexual fitness. For more complete information, you should purchase a book specifically dedicated to the topic or speak with your physician. There is an excellent and comprehensive (but also highly clinical because its target audience is doctors) reference text by Dr. Theresa Crenshaw and Dr. James Goldberg called *Sexual Pharmacology: Drugs That Affect Sexual Function*.

To give you a better idea of how drugs can have an impact on sexual fitness, we'll take an in-depth look at two categories of prescription medications: antihypertensives and antidepressants. These drugs are widely used and also have well-researched sexual side effects.

Antihypertensives

Antihypertensives are used to treat high blood pressure. Most people, once they begin taking the medication, continue to take it for the rest of their lives. As a result, antihypertensives are some of the most prescribed medications in the United States today. They are also commonly recognized as being detrimental to sexual function.

Because antihypertensives lower blood pressure, in effect they decrease blood flow to the genital region. Decades of research prove that this increases the rates of erectile and ejaculatory dysfunction in men. In addition, antihypertensives cause a drop in levels of certain sex hormones, which can result in decreased sexual desire in both men and women.

However, if you take antihypertensives, you need not despair. Diuretics, beta-blockers, alpha-blockers, and alpha-antagonists appear to most hinder sexual performance and enjoyment. As an alternative to these drugs, consider asking your doctor about more recent antihypertensive medications: ACE inhibitors and calcium channel blockers. While these drugs can still have a negative impact on erections due to lowered blood pressure, they appear to be a significant improvement over the other options in terms of overall sexual enjoyment.

Antidepressants

Depression is a serious and surprisingly common illness. Depression itself can be devastating to sexuality, usually affecting desire the most, but often interfering with sexual performance as well. Antidepressants work miraculously for many people, alleviating their overwhelming feelings of futility, sadness, fatigue, and irritation and restoring their enthusiasm for life. Yet some types of antidepressants, including tricyclics, monoamine oxidase inhibitors (MAOIs), and selective serotonin reuptake inhibitors (SSRIs), can have a serious impact on libido and sexual pleasure even if the depression is adequately treated.

SSRIs are the most commonly used antidepressants in the U.S. These drugs, which are sold under the brand names of Prozac, Zoloft, and Paxil, work by increasing levels of the neurotransmitter serotonin in the brain. Although serotonin very effectively combats depression, unfortunately it also inhibits sexual desire and orgasm and delays ejaculation.

If you take an SSRI-class of antidepressant and believe that it has interfered with your sex life, speak with your doctor. Please do consult your physician before taking any course of action. You might be able to switch to a different type of antidepressant. For example, Wellbutrin (bupropion) is considered to have little or no effect on sexual function and is therefore labeled "sex friendly."

With your doctor's approval, you might also try switching away from your prescription medication to a natural supplement called St. John's wort (*Hypericum perforatum*). Repeated clinical trials have demonstrated that an extract made of this flowering plant is just as effective as standard antidepressants in treating depression, but with fewer side effects. Specifically, the herb does not appear to have any negative impact on sexuality.

SEXUAL SIDE EFFECTS OF SOME COMMON MEDICATIONS

DRUG CATEGORY	COMMON BRAND NAMES	POTENTIAL NEGATIVE SEXUAL SIDE EFFECTS	ALTERNATIVES
Antihypertensives that are diuretics, reserpine, methyldopa, guanethidine, beta-blockers, alpha-blockers, or alpha antagonists	• Hygroton • Hydrodiuril • Serpasil • Aldomet • Ismelin • Inderal • Tenormin • Catapres	• Erectile dysfunction • Ejaculatory dysfunction • Decreased desire • Infertility (beta-blockers only)	Antihypertensives that are ACE inhibitors (e.g., Vasotec, Capoten) or calcium channel blockers (e.g., Cardizem, Calan) appear to be the least sexually disruptive.
Asthma medications	• Bronkaid Mist • Primatene Mist • Atrovent	• Nervousness and irritability lead to decreased desire • Decreased testosterone production (corticosteroids only) • Vaginal dryness (anti-cholinergics only)	Asthma medications that are beta antagonists (Proventil, Ventolin) appear to be the least sexually disruptive.
Anti-ulcer drugs	• Zantac • Pepcid • Axid • Tagamet	• Breast sensitivity • Erectile dysfunction • Infertility (cimetidine only) • Desire disorders (cimetidine only)	Antiulcer drugs made of ranitidine (Zantac), famotidine (Pepcid), and nizatidine (Axid) appear to be less sexually disruptive than cimetidine (Tagamet)

Antidepressants that are tricyclics, MAOIs, and SSRIs	• Anafranil • Elavil • Marplan • Nardil • Prozac • Zoloft • Paxil • Luvox	• Desire disorders • Erectile dysfunction • Ejaculatory disorders • Menstrual disorders • Fertility disorders (tricyclics only) • Orgasm difficulties • Breast disorders	Antidepressants made of bupropion (Wellbutrin) appear to be significantly less sexually disruptive.
Cold/Allergy medications that are antihistamines or contain pseudoephedrine	• Chlor-Trimeton • Benadryl • Excedrin PM • Sudafed	• Drowsiness • Vaginal dryness • Erectile difficulties	Noticeable sexual side effects should only occur with chronic use.
Birth control pills that are monophasic	• Ortho-Novum 1/35 • Norinyl 1+35 • Brevicon • Modicon • Ovcon 35	• Decreased libido • Vaginal dryness • Orgasm difficulties	Birth control pills that are triphasic (Ortho Tri-Cyclen, Tri-Norinyl, Ortho Novum 7/7/7) or contain levonorgestrel (Nordette, Levlen) have zero to few sexual side effects.
Antianxiety agents that are benzodiazepines	• Xanax • Valium • Ativan • Librium • Restoril	• Decreased libido • Orgasm difficulties • Erection disorders • Ejaculation disorders	Antianxiety medications that contain buspirone (BuSpar) appear to have the fewest sexual side effects.

If you must remain on your current antidepressants, doctors recommend some helpful strategies for reducing their impact on your sex life. You might be able to take a lower dose of the drug. You can also try to have sex in the morning before you take your medication, when levels of the drug in your body are lowest. Finally, your doctor might allow you to take "drug holidays": you stop taking your medication before and during a romantic getaway for a few days in order to optimize your sex drive.

It is important to remember that your health comes first. If you need to take medications, there are frequently ways to deal with the sexual side effects. After all, having sex isn't going to do you much good in the face of a heart attack! At the same time, you may want to visit your doctor if you have any doubts or concerns about how the drugs you take may be affecting your sexuality. Be proactive and approach your physician openly with your questions. Many people may feel embarrassed to discuss sexual concerns with their doctors, and doctors may neglect to bring up the fact that medications have sexual side effects. Yet you can overcome these barriers by expressing what is on your mind and asking your specific questions. Don't be shy. Whatever you do, please don't simply stop taking your medication. You will definitely need professional guidance in determining how best to adapt your medication regimen to optimize your sexual fitness and overall health.

Hormones

Hormones occur naturally in the body and play a crucial role in sexual function. They are responsible for sexual differences between men and women. They govern many aspects of human sexuality including sexual thoughts and dreams, the urge to have sex, genital arousal (vaginal lubrication and genital engorgement in women and penile erection in men), and the ability to reach orgasm. Hormones are also essential to reproduction: they regulate the menstrual cycle and ovulation in women, and sperm production in men.

Hormone levels constantly vary depending on the time of day and month, your general health, what medications you're taking, and many other factors. Levels of hormones also tend to drop as we age, quickly for women during menopause and more gradually for men (a controversial phenomenon called male menopause or "andropause"). These changes in hormone levels can have a dramatic impact on sexual desire and pleasure.

As a result of this natural hormonal decline, one-third of menopausal women in the United States and a growing number of men choose to take hormones in the form of prescription medication. This treatment, known as hormone replacement therapy (HRT), boosts diminishing hormone levels in order to combat negative health effects (such as hot flashes and osteoporosis in women) as well as to restore libido and sexual function.

While HRT can prove beneficial, specifically to those suffering from a hormone deficiency, the decision to use these powerful drugs should not be taken lightly. Hormones can have a powerful impact on sexuality as well as general health and wellness. But we are only just beginning to fully understand the subtle and long-term effects of hormone supplementation on our minds and bodies.

Estrogen

Estrogen is considered the female sex hormone because it causes female sexual characteristics to emerge during neonatal development. It plays a critical role in the menstrual cycle and consequent ovulation and fertility, and is a key ingredient in many birth control pills. It also allows vaginal lubrication to occur in response to sexual arousal.

However, estrogen does not appear to have an impact on sex drive—testosterone contributes most to libido in both men and women.

When women lack adequate amounts of estrogen, either due to menopause, oopherectomy (surgical removal of the ovaries), or other health reasons, they may experience vaginal dryness and thinning of the vaginal walls. This frequently results in pain during intercourse, directly interfering with sexual pleasure. Estrogen replacement therapy (ERT) effectively reduces these symptoms by restoring vaginal wall thickness and the ability of the genital tissues to undergo vasocongestion (dilation of the blood vessels), which leads to lubrication.

For many women, estrogen loss has its biggest impact on sexual fitness in terms of general mood and state of mind. Clinical research consistently finds that ERT improves women's sense of well-being. ERT can control hot flashes, irritability, depression, and mood swings. In two European studies, postmenopausal women using an estrogen patch reported improved quality of life and sex life.

However, there are some risks. ERT can cause spotty, menstrual-like bleeding, and even symptoms that resemble PMS. Increasing estrogen levels can also cause a corresponding drop in testosterone, which may contribute to loss of libido. In order to combat this decrease in sex drive, doctors may recommend adding testosterone to ERT. Testosterone supplementation comes with its own set of issues, which we'll discuss later in the chapter. Finally, ERT may increase the risk of breast cancer, although this issue is hotly debated in the scientific community and no consensus has yet been reached.

Progesterone

Progesterone is another female hormone. It gets its name from the fact that it aids in gestation—helping the implantation of the fertilized egg and the maintenance of the fetus during pregnancy. It also acts as a natural contraceptive by preventing ovulation and is therefore a key ingredient (sometimes the only hormone) in birth control pills.

Progesterone is frequently included in HRT. Women on estrogen must take progesterone as well in order to minimize their risk of uterine cancer. (The exception is if a woman has had a hysterectomy, in which case she has no uterus and therefore uterine cancer is not a risk.) Progesterone may also play a role in the maintenance of bones and in helping to reduce hot flashes.

In large doses, progesterone may cause loss of libido, mood swings, weight gain, and PMS-like complaints. However, most birth control pills and HRT today contain very small doses, which should have minimal side effects. One risk to consider: A recent study published in the *Journal of the American Medical Association* suggested that estrogen-progesterone therapy might increase the risk of breast cancer more than estrogen treatment alone.

These factors make undergoing HRT a complex decision. It may be the best option for some women but not for others. Women with menopausal complaints should carefully consider their choices along with their doctors.

Testosterone

Androgens—testosterone and androstenedione—are the primary sex hormones in men. They are responsible for male secondary sex characteristics, such as a low voice and facial hair, as well as sexual function and fertility. Later in life, testosterone is responsible for the biological drive or "urge" to have sex in both men and women.

Testosterone is often called the male sex hormone because it is found naturally in higher concentrations in men than in women. However, it is responsible for libido, sexual thoughts and fantasy, and frequency of sexual activity in both genders. There is no doubt that testosterone is linked to sexual impulses. The efficacy and value of testosterone replacement therapy (TRT) in improving sexual function, however, is up for debate. Since both natural levels of testosterone and effects of TRT vary greatly by gender, we'll discuss men and women separately.

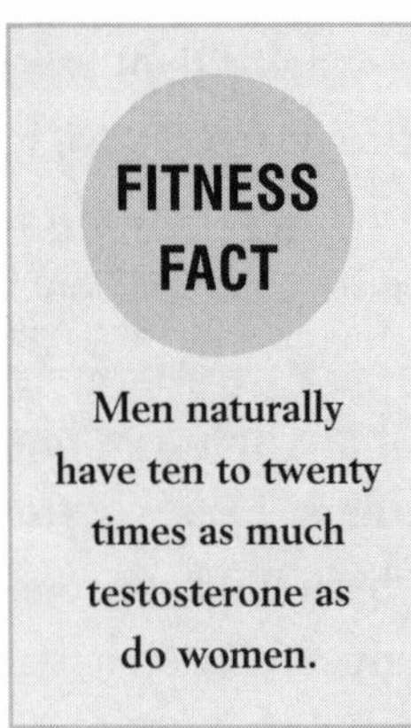

Men naturally have ten to twenty times as much testosterone as do women.

TESTOSTERONE IN MEN Between the ages of forty-five and fifty, men's testosterone levels naturally begin to decline. For certain individuals, this reduction can have a significant impact on sexual fitness. If their testosterone levels are abnormally low, men will first experience a drop in libido and eventually have difficulty reaching orgasm. When they do reach orgasm, the volume of ejaculate may be smaller. Low testosterone levels may result in impaired fertility. In addition, lack of testosterone may decrease muscle strength and stamina and bring on depressivelike symptoms.

TRT has proven highly effective in restoring sexual function for men with low testosterone levels. Clear evidence for the benefits of TRT comes from tests conducted on men who have had their testes, the primary source of testosterone, either physically removed or totally suppressed by chemicals. When they are treated with testosterone, these men rapidly regain their interest in sex and ability to ejaculate. Aging men whose testosterone levels are naturally declining respond similarly well to TRT.

A few warnings, though: First, TRT does not help overcome erectile dysfunction. Even though ED is common in men over fifty, this problem is not entirely dependent on hormonal status. Men who are testosterone deficient have occasional erections even when they have no sexual appetite. Also, men with already normal to high testosterone levels will not benefit from TRT. In other words, increasing testosterone above average levels does not provide any added benefits, and can result in side effects such as reduced sperm count, prostate enlargement, and liver damage.

Since low sex drive does not necessarily mean testosterone deficiency, doctors will usually test your testosterone levels when you complain of libido loss. Responsible physicians will recommend TRT only if your testosterone levels are abnormally low. If you decide to go forward with TRT, make sure that your doctor carefully monitors your progress.

TESTOSTERONE IN WOMEN Testosterone is the hormone responsible for the biological component of sex drive in women as well as in men. Women with medium to high testosterone levels report greater sexual arousal, more masturbation, and a higher frequency of sexual dreams than women with low testosterone levels do. The hormone also contributes to a positive mood and overall sense of well-being. Abnormally low testosterone levels, on the other hand, can lead to a lack of sexual interest, decreased sexual pleasure, difficulty with orgasm, and sometimes depression.

A common complaint of many postmenopausal women is that they simply no longer desire sexual intimacy, and one of the reasons for this may be their lowered testosterone levels. However, depression, poor sexual experiences (pain during intercourse, lack of pleasure, or a partner's ED), ill health, and relationship difficulties can also contribute to lack of sexual passion. It may be tempting to rush into your doctor's office and request TRT thinking "Surely this will be the answer!" But if an abnormally low testosterone level is not the major contributing cause of your lowered libido in the first place, the results of TRT will likely be disappointing.

That having been said, menopause does cause testosterone levels to plummet to about half premenopausal levels. For some women, especially those who had higher than average levels of testosterone prior to menopause, this drop will be keenly felt. TRT may be their best option. In numerous clinical studies, menopausal women with low testosterone levels report increased libido and sexual responsiveness when given small doses of testosterone.

TRT is also effective for women who have had their ovaries removed (an oopherectomy, which may be done during a hysterectomy). Nearly 50 percent of women report a loss of libido and other sexual dysfunction after having this procedure because in females the ovaries are primarily responsible for testosterone production. When given TRT, most of these women report a significant boost to their sex drive, arousal levels, and frequency of sexual fantasy.

Although research into TRT for women is still in its early stages, there appear to be some concerns and controversies with long-term treatment. The debate centers on the effects of testosterone on cholesterol and the risk of developing hormone-related cancers (e.g., breast and uterine).

However, doctors are increasingly willing to prescribe TRT to menopausal women who have abnormally low testosterone levels. To date, it appears that testosterone should only be taken in combination with ERT and not alone. You should make an informed decision about whether or not to try this approach only after careful consideration of your medical history, general health, and specific concerns with your doctor.

DHEA

Dehydroepiandrosterone (DHEA) is the newest piece of the hormone puzzle. It is converted to estrogen and testosterone in the body and is therefore known as a "prohormone." Levels of DHEA steadily decline throughout adulthood. Studies suggest that DHEA supplementation can improve overall sense of well-being, inhibit osteoporosis, and stimulate weight loss for people with low levels of the prohormone.

DHEA appears to play a critical role in sexual vitality. For men, it is involved in erectile function. A study published the *Journal of Urology* revealed that as DHEA levels fall, incidence of ED increases. In women, DHEA seems to affect sexual drive and pleasure. One clinical trial found that supplementation with the prohormone effectively raised testosterone levels, increased sexual interest and frequency of sexual thoughts, and enhanced sexual satisfaction among a group of women with low DHEA levels.

FITNESS FACT

By the age of sixty, people have less than one-third as much DHEA in their bodies as they did at age twenty.

Despite these promising signs, it's important to exercise caution when considering DHEA supplementation. Clinical trials are still limited, and most of those have been short-term tests conducted on animals or small numbers of people. Preliminary research indicates that DHEA may raise cholesterol levels, cause liver damage, and increase the risk of certain types of cancer. Because of the current lack of scientific knowledge, many doctors advise against the use of DHEA at this time.

Androstenedione

Androstenedione is, like DHEA, a prohormone. It is naturally converted to testosterone in the body. Among women over forty, high levels of androstenedione are correlated with high levels of sexual interest and arousal. Manufacturers, who sell the powerful prohormone as a natural supplement called "andro," claim that it can enhance sex drive and performance.

However, there is no evidence that taking andro supplements will increase testosterone levels or have an impact on sexual function. In a clinical trial, andro treatment did nothing to improve sexual passion in a group of women suffering from low libido. Aside from being ineffective, andro also has serious potential health risks, including increased risk of heart, prostate, and liver problems. With prolonged use, men may experience erectile dysfunction and women may develop

POTENTIAL EFFECTS OF HORMONE SUPPLEMENTATION—SUMMARY

HORMONE	PURPOSE OF TREATMENT	SEXUAL FITNESS ADVANTAGES	DISADVANTAGES
Estrogen	For women with low estrogen levels or suffering from menopausal symptoms	• Improves vaginal lubrication • Prevents thinning of vaginal walls • Reduces pain during intercourse • Decreases anxiety, depression, and irritability	• Produces PMS-like symptoms • May cause loss of libido • May increase risk of breast cancer
Progesterone	For women on estrogen replacement therapy (ERT)	• Must be taken with estrogen to reduce risk of uterine cancer • May reduce hot flashes	• Produces PMS-like symptoms • May increase risk of breast cancer
Testosterone—Men	For men with low testosterone levels	• Increases sexual motivation, arousal, and fantasy • Enables ejaculation • Enhances mood and improves sense of well-being	• Suppresses sperm production • Encourages prostate growth • Can cause liver damage

Testosterone—Women	For women with low testosterone levels or on ERT	• Increases sexual motivation, arousal, and fantasy • Increases ease of attaining orgasm • Improves sexual responsiveness • Enhances mood and improves sense of well-being	• Increases cholesterol levels • May cause liver damage • May increase risk of breast and uterine cancers
DHEA	For men and women with low DHEA levels	• Increases sexual interest, fantasy, and satisfaction • Reduces erectile dysfunction • Enhances mood and improves sense of well-being	• May increase cholesterol levels, cause liver damage, and increase cancer risk • Long-term effects have not been researched and are not well understood
Andro	For people who want to improve their sexual drive and performance	• Claims to boost sex drive and performance	• No evidence for purported advantages • Leads to male characteristics (e.g., deep voice and facial hair) in women • Prolonged use causes ED in men • May cause heart, prostate, and liver problems • Long-term effects have not been researched and are not well understood

masculine-type characteristics such as lowered voice, facial hair, and decreased breast size.

Now let's take a brief look at some prosexual drugs—prescription pharmaceuticals designed specifically for the treatment of sexual dysfunction. Most people are probably familiar with Viagra, which has received a great deal of press coverage. Aside from Viagra and the hormonal therapies just discussed in the previous section, there are several other products currently on the market, as well. However, we shall focus on Viagra, as it is the most probable treatment for a vast majority of men suffering from erectile dysfunction today.

Viagra (scientific name *sildenafil citrate*) is the first FDA-approved prescription pill for the treatment of ED. Since its release in March 1998, the drug has exploded in popularity, becoming one of the most successful prescription pharmaceuticals ever launched. It has also brought the issue of ED out into the open for millions of men and women around the world. For the first time, people feel a bit more comfortable walking into their doctors' offices and bringing up the sensitive topic of sexual difficulties.

There is no question that Viagra works for many men who suffer from the partial or total inability to achieve and maintain an erection. Viagra is very specific in its action on the body. It works to keep nitric oxide from being broken down. When nitric oxide is plentiful, the blood vessels of the penis can relax and ample amounts of blood can flow into the erectile tissue. Within an hour of taking Viagra—with proper sexual stimulation—users can enjoy stronger and longer-lasting erections. Some men experience improved ability for extended periods of time: they may even see the return of long-lost morning erections the night after taking the pill.

However, men need to be able to produce nitric oxide in the first place in order for Viagra to work. Since nitric oxide comes from the nerve endings, lining of the blood vessels, and smooth muscle cells of the penis, Viagra will not work as well for men who have inadequate sources of nitric oxide (i.e., due to nerve damage from surgery, diabetes, injury to the blood vessel lining from hypertension, and smoking). This also explains why Viagra does not work if a man is not aroused. When he's not stimulated, his body won't produce nitric oxide; and if he doesn't produce nitric oxide, Viagra cannot help.

So far, Viagra has been proven effective only for men, and its potential benefits for women are as yet unclear. Though subject to major debate, some scientists theorize that if Viagra can enhance erections in men, it may have similar effects for women with impaired blood flow to their erectile tissues. Whether Viagra might enhance vaginal lubrication, ease of orgasm, and other female sexual functions is not known.

Viagra does have troublesome side effects for some users, including headaches, stuffy nose, flushing, stomach upset, and, rarely, blue-tinted vision. Viagra itself does not cause heart attacks. However, men who have heart disease or congestive heart failure that requires the use of any form of nitroglycerine, or men who cannot tolerate the physical exertion of sex itself, are advised not to take the drug because of the risk. Viagra is also not recommended for men who are on certain antihypertensive medications. It should be used with caution in combination with other prescription drugs that may alter its level in the blood or delay its clearance out of the system.

Bill is a man who has recently discovered the benefits of Viagra. Bill has had diabetes since he was fifteen years old. He remembers being devastated with the diagnosis at the time. He thought it meant that he wouldn't be able to play baseball with his friends and would be ostracized at school. But after some time, he discovered that diabetes was something he could live with, that he could still have the happy life he'd always wanted. He married his high school sweetheart, Chloe, and had three healthy children by the time he was twenty-seven years of age. He felt he had a strong and sexually satisfying relationship with his wife.

But then things slowly began to change. By the time he was thirty-five, Bill began experiencing difficulties with his erections. Over the years, the problem grew worse. By age sixty, he couldn't maintain an erection firm enough to have intercourse with Chloe. After a while, he and Chloe stopped making love. They adapted to the situation and decided that they could live with a very low level of sexual intimacy.

Then one day at the diabetic clinic Bill picked up a pamphlet about Viagra. Right away, he wanted to try it. Although his doctor explained that the success rate was lower for diabetics, he agreed that Bill should give it a try.

Bill started with the recommended dose of Viagra. He and his wife went out for a fancy dinner and he took the little blue pill as the meal ended. They were both pretty excited and began making love as soon as they arrived home, but Bill's erection was a disappointment. It was still not firm enough for intercourse. Nevertheless, Bill and Chloe felt motivated to try again another day. Bill's doctor recommended that he increase the dose to the maximum level. When he did, Bill found that his erections were adequate for penetration. Bill feels grateful that he and Chloe now have the option to enjoy lovemaking again.

The FDA has approved several other drugs for ED—MUSE, Caverject, and Edex—which are based on using other methods to enhance erectile function. These products rely on prostaglandin to cause the muscles of the penile blood vessels to relax, thereby initiating erections. These medications have proved effective for some men in clinical trials. They are a good alternative for patients who do not respond to or cannot take Viagra. The major disadvantage of these products is that they need to be applied directly to the penile tissue. Caverject or Edex must be injected into the side of the penis, and MUSE must be inserted into the urethra.

Newer-generation prosexual drugs are on their way. These products will try to eliminate some of the problems with Viagra. What's more, research into drugs designed specifically to address female sexual dysfunction is just starting to increase. But it's not necessary for you to wait for more drugs to be developed in order to improve your sexual passion, pleasure, and performance. You can begin to take control of your sexual vitality and overall health by starting the Sexual Fitness Program today!

Other Influences on Your Sexual Health

Although technically not considered medication, nicotine, alcohol, and caffeine are indulgences that many people use to medicate themselves. Most of us enjoy a glass of wine or a cup of coffee from time to time, and achieving sexual fitness does not require giving up these indulgences completely. However, it's important to keep in mind that anything harmful to your body, mind, and general health can also be harmful to your sexual wellness. When you choose to take control of your substance consumption, you reduce the obstacles between you and sexual fulfillment.

Let's take a look at the effects that cigarettes, alcohol, and caffeine have on sexual fitness. A great deal of research has been done on the health consequences of these substances. Many of these studies examine the impact of heavy, long-term abuse. In every case, real addiction to a drug can cause infertility, ED, loss of libido, or all of the above. That having been said, moderate consumption of alcohol and caffeine does not appear to harm sexual fitness, and may even have limited benefits. Read on to find out what the research says we can consider "safe" dosages of certain substances, and which ones you're better off eliminating from your life altogether.

Nicotine

Smoking cigarettes is disastrous for your health. This is no surprise. We've all read the research and heard about the multibillion-dollar lawsuits. Here's a brief review of the facts, just in case you need a reminder: Smokers have far higher mortality rates than do nonsmokers. They are also at greater risk for lung cancer, emphysema, heart attack, stroke, and many other medical problems. In addition, smoking is devastating to sexual fitness—it leads to ED and infertility.

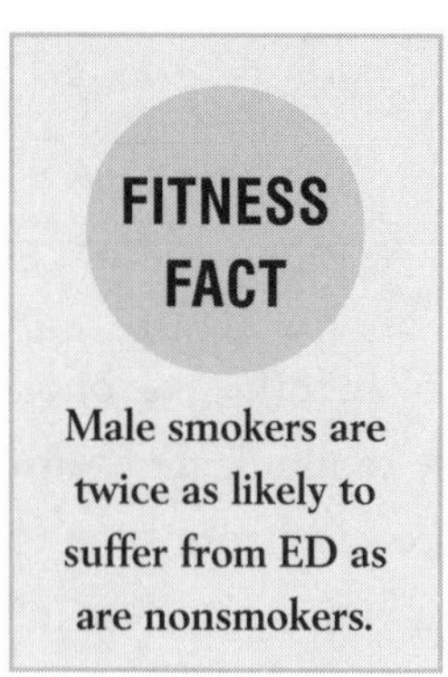

Male smokers are twice as likely to suffer from ED as are nonsmokers.

Smoking causes impotence by restricting circulation. Erections depend on blood flowing into the delicate arteries of the penis and filling the erectile tissue. When blood flow is inadequate, erections cannot occur.

Little research has been done to examine the effects of smoking on female sexual arousal. However, optimum female sexual pleasure also depends upon adequate blood flow to the genital region. Like the penis, the clitoris and vagina become engorged with blood during arousal. Therefore, smoking most likely interferes with female sexual function by restricting circulation, as it does in men.

Smoking creates an imbalance in hormone levels and thereby interferes with normal menstrual cycles, as well. Female smokers have a higher prevalence of irregular or infrequent menstrual cycles and early menopause than nonsmokers do. In fact, moderate smokers (fewer than twenty cigarettes per day) experience 20 percent more frequent abnormal vaginal bleeding than expected, and heavy smokers (more than twenty cigarettes per day) experience 67 percent more.

If you smoke, here's a great incentive to finally kick the habit: Your sexual fitness depends upon your quitting. Regardless of whether you are old or young, male or female, a recent smoker or a lifetime addict, your sexual vitality and overall health will improve when you quit. You will feel better, look better, taste and smell better to your lover, appear more attractive, and enjoy better sex.

Alcohol

For centuries, people have used alcohol to stimulate their sex drive. In moderate quantities, it can reduce anxiety and release us from social inhibitions. However, alcohol is a sedative, and after more than one or two drinks, the body begins to feel its effects and performance can suffer. Scientific studies reveal that alcohol generally enhances *psychological* arousal but inhibits *physiological* arousal.

From a psychological perspective, alcohol can act as a sexual aid by inducing feelings of calm and relaxation. When we're less anxious, we're also more likely to be in the mood for sex. Moreover, drinking triggers learned expectations: we expect alcohol to make us more amorous, and therefore it does. As people's blood alcohol levels increase, so does their self-reported arousal—at the same time as their physical ability to enjoy sex is declining.

From a physiological perspective, consuming one to two drinks may have a slightly positive impact on sexual fitness, but more than that will only do you harm. As you begin to ingest alcohol, your body increases its production of dopamine, the neurotransmitter most closely linked to libido and sexual enjoyment. You may therefore experience a sexual boost after one or two drinks. Also, alcohol acts as a vasodilator, increasing blood flow throughout the body. So having a couple of drinks may actually enhance erections and vaginal arousal.

As your level of intoxication increases, however, alcohol begins to interfere with arousal and orgasm. Sex hormone levels decline, which can interfere with libido and performance. With every additional drink, men have more and more difficulty maintaining an erection and ejaculating. One study found that it took men significantly more time to reach orgasm after three to four drinks than when they were sober, and after heavy alcohol consumption many subjects were unable to ejaculate at all. Female sexual performance also suffers. Vaginal blood flow, lubrication, and orgasmic intensity are all impaired after just a few drinks. One study revealed that the time it took women to reach orgasm while masturbating increased each time their blood alcohol levels rose. With no alcohol it took them an average of about six minutes to climax, but after consuming four to five drinks, the average time to reach orgasm was about fourteen minutes.

Alcoholism causes permanent damage to sexual fitness. It reduces testosterone levels, which results in loss of desire for both men and women. And it damages the nervous system, thereby interfering with sexual response and pleasure. There is a high rate of erectile dysfunction among male alcoholics. Female alcoholics typically suffer from abnormal menstruation and infertility.

On the whole, heavy alcohol consumption (4 or more drinks per day) can be devastating to your sexual health. Light (0 to 2 drinks per day) alcohol consumption may have some benefits, but this requires maintaining control and not overdoing it. In order to optimize your sexual fitness, you should drink no more than one to two glasses of alcohol a day on a regular basis.

Caffeine

Caffeine is the most widely used drug in the world today. If you're one of the many people with this daily habit, here's a piece of good news: You don't have to quit. In fact, as caffeine serves to arouse the nervous system, boost the metabolic rate, and increase blood flow, moderate consumption (defined as two cups or about 200 to 300 mg per day) may offer some benefits to sexual fitness. A small study of older men indicated that coffee enhanced their sex lives by providing them with extra energy.

However, you should limit your intake to no more than two cups of coffee or four cans of caffeinated soda a day. At doses any higher than that, caffeine can alter levels of sex hormones and may cause some serious physical and psychological problems. For women, heavy caffeine intake is associated with a significantly increased risk of ovar-

CAFFEINE CONTENT OF SOME COMMON DRINKS*	
Brewed coffee	100–150 mg
Instant coffee	40–108 mg
Brewed tea	9–46 mg
Instant tea	12–28 mg
Decaffeinated coffee	2–5 mg
Most caffeinated colas	36–55 mg

*Five-ounce cup/12-ounce can.

ian cancer and endometriosis. Also, studies indicate that caffeine intake is correlated with severity of PMS symptoms: the more caffeine women consume, the worse the PMS. In both men and women, heavy caffeine consumption can cause anxiety, restlessness, nervousness, insomnia, lack of focus, and gastrointestinal disturbances.

The bottom line for caffeine drinkers is moderation. It seems that consuming fewer than two cups of coffee or four cans of soda a day will do you no harm, and it may just give you a needed energy boost at times when you're feeling too tired to play. However, once you exceed that limit, you put yourself at risk for health problems. So enjoy your daily dose of caffeine, but remember to take it easy.

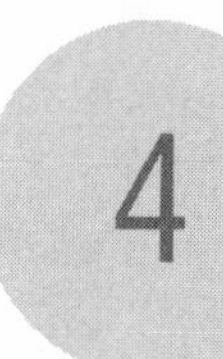

Sensual Stimulation

> Various types of nourishing and savory foods and sweet, delicious, refreshing drinks, a conversation which is pleasing to the ears and a light touch which caresses the skin, clear nights, which are sweetened by the rays of a full moon . . . pleasant songs, which entrance and captivate the soul, the chewing of betel leaves, wine and garlands, wound from sweetly scented flowers, and a happy and unencumbered heart—these are the best aphrodisiacs in life.
>
> —SUSRATA, INDIAN SURGEON, 800 B.C.

When most of us think of lovemaking, it is first of the physical act: Two bodies joining together. When you hear the word *sex*, what comes to mind is the response of your body as it is aroused; the sensations you feel as your lover caresses you; the physical pleasure of orgasm.

Yet sex involves all the senses, not just physical touch. Complete sensual stimulation leads to the most erotic and fulfilling experiences. With all your senses actively involved, you can lose yourself to passionate intimacy. In a positive sexual experience, the entire universe seems to encompass only you and your lover. You look into your partner's eyes and experience a connection that reaches into the very depths of your soul. You feel your bodies entwine. You hear the sounds of both your breaths. You smell the sweet scent of perfume and cologne mixed with sweat. You taste your lover's salty lips.

When all the senses are involved, not only does the sexual

experience become richer, but you also find yourself more excited about and engaged in what is taking place because you are fully present and sensually aware. By stimulating your senses, you make use of all the wonderful tools that your body has to offer and enable yourself to reach a whole new level of lovemaking.

Melissa and Karl have found that integrating sensual stimulation into their lives has contributed greatly to their sexuality. Both of them are in their mid-thirties and in excellent health. They work out regularly, eat a nutritious diet, and have no major health concerns. However, as the parents of two young children, they often find themselves too busy and too tired for sex. They work during the day, take care of their kids in the mornings and evenings, and fill their weekends with family activities. They find that by the time they hit the sack, they're in no mood for romance. "If you're running around all day feeling stressed out, you can't just go straight to sex," says Melissa.

In order to make sexual intimacy a priority in their lives again, Melissa and Karl decided to try paying attention to their senses—focusing on sensuality rather than sex, per se. "The simple things worked the best for us: massage, candles, and baths," they confided later. "The point for us is to make time to get in touch with each other. Planning for these activities really made a difference."

After Melissa and Karl put the children to bed, the first step they take is to light several aromatherapy candles. "Candlelight is more romantic," Melissa says. "Plus, as soon as I smell them, I feel instantly relaxed. Also, lighting candles just gives us time to wind down. It serves as a transition from our hectic day to our peaceful, intimate time alone." Such a small act as this often serves as a signal for the pleasurable experiences to come.

Next, they settle down in bed and exchange massages. These massages sometimes last a half hour, but usually they're just five to ten minutes long. "If you expect massages to be long and involved, then you won't do them as often," explains Melissa. "By keeping them short, we find time to do them several times a week."

Melissa finds that massages really help her get in the mood. "It stimulates me. When I'm stressed, all my nerve endings shut off. Someone can touch me and I don't feel anything. Massage turns my nerve endings back on. It makes me feel alive again. And then the sex is much better because I'm feeling sensation all over my body instead of only in the genital area. It makes orgasms so much better."

Sometimes Melissa and Karl will share a bath, but this usually happens only on weekends or special occasions because of the time commitment involved. They light a few candles in the bathroom, turn off the lights, play soft music, and relax in the warm, scented water. When they're done, Melissa says, she feels sexy and happy.

All in all, Melissa and Karl are very pleased with their sensual habits. "They take so little time and effort," Melissa explains emphatically, "and the benefit is so great. This is the best thing we could've done for our sex life."

When you make use of the activities and follow the recommendations provided in this chapter, you should notice a new level of enthusiasm and sexual enjoyment right away. Sensual stimulation actually works on both the psychological and physiological levels to increase arousal and intensify the sexual experience. These positive changes will inspire you to keep up with the rest of your Sexual Fitness Program by serving as a reminder that you are working to improve your sexual passion and pleasure every day.

Touch

The healing power of human touch binds us together into families and communities and encourages intimacy. No single sense contributes as much to sexual pleasure as does touch. When we're initially attracted to someone, we feel our skin tingle and our hearts throb. Lovemaking is dominated by touch, two bodies joining together. The physical sensations of kissing, caressing, penetrating, and engulfing are the very essence of the sexual act. Touch gives us the most intense ecstasy we can experience.

Touch directly serves to enhance sexual fitness by stimulating the secretion of oxytocin, a hormone that induces a state of pleasure and provides a sense of satiation. Oxytocin levels are naturally highest in men and women during sexual arousal and peak during orgasm. Oxytocin encourages bonding between sexual partners, fostering feelings of love and friendship. It enhances sexual interest, fantasy, and desire for intercourse. Oxytocin also appears to have a direct impact on sexual performance by facilitating orgasm and improving erectile function. Please note that hormones do not work alone, and several dozen chemicals can combine in various ways to produce any given effect. Nevertheless, oxytocin clearly has a profound effect on sexual behavior and enjoyment.

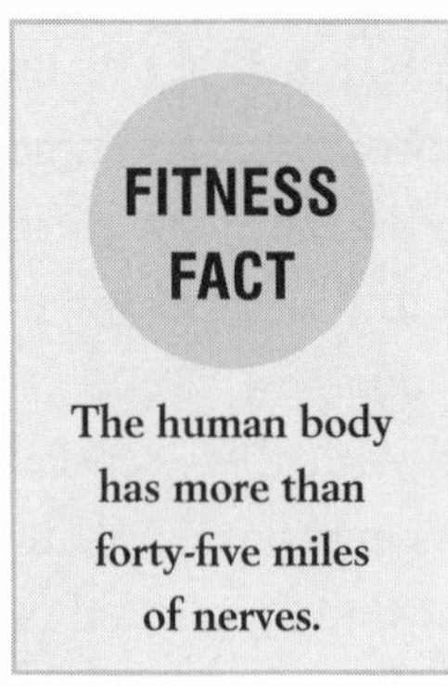

You can naturally stimulate the release of oxytocin by making optimum use of your sense of touch. Studies show that gentle touch in the form of massage, hugging and kissing, and physical closeness facilitates oxytocin production. So do warm temperatures in the form of a bath, cuddling with your lover, or snuggling under a blanket.

In addition, stimulating the genital region and other erogenous zones, either through masturbation or sexual activity with a partner, causes oxytocin levels to rise. This increase does not occur due to arousal alone. In a clinical trial involving men and women, viewing sexually explicit material did not result in an oxytocin boost. However, once subjects were allowed to stimulate themselves, oxytocin levels rose steadily, soaring to the highest levels with orgasm. This relationship among oxytocin, physical stimulation, and orgasm illustrates how important touch is to the human sexual experience.

Touch Tips

Now that you know how touch influences sexual fitness, let's move on to how you can take full advantage of this magnificent sense. Below, you'll find tips for using touch to enhance your own and your partner's sexual pleasure and performance.

1. Maintain your body's testosterone production.

Androgens (the so-called male sex hormones, which includes testosterone) appear to be at least partially responsible for making touch feel sexual. When our androgen levels are abnormally low, we enjoy less sensitivity to touch and our bodies do not interpret touch stimuli as sexual.

If you are over fifty and suffering from sexual dysfunction, postmenopausal and experiencing low libido, or diabetic, you may have below-average testosterone levels; and this may be interfering with your ability to perceive touch in a sexual way. Although testosterone replacement therapy (TRT) is an option for some groups of people (see chapter 3: *Substances*), the truth is that most of us should benefit from a gentle, natural approach to maintaining testosterone in our bodies. As you have seen in these first few chapters, treating your body well by following the Sexual Fitness Program can have a positive impact on your hormone levels.

2. Explore sexual activity without intercourse or orgasm as your goal.

In our society, reaching orgasm often becomes the sole focus of sex. This unnecessary pressure can create performance anxiety and interfere with sexual pleasure for both men and women.

Sex therapists sometimes treat anxiety and other sexual problems but still encourage intimacy and pleasure by asking couples to explore touch without expectations of either orgasm or sexual intercourse. In this way, couples can learn to refocus their attention from performance (having an erect penis, reaching orgasm) to connecting with each other and feeling good. As a result of their new relaxed attitudes, sex therapists report, the partners frequently learn to enjoy heightened levels of sexual understanding and enjoyment.

3. Practice nonsexual touch.

Nonsexual touch means stroking, hugging, kissing, and rubbing your partner without intending sexual activity. There are many benefits to nonsexual touch. It can help build intimacy, further stimulate your sex drive by making you hold off for the reward, enhance awareness of your body, create greater intimacy through trust and security, and remind you of the many joys of simple physical closeness. Couples who don't touch except to have sex miss out on the full spectrum of what sexual intimacy can be.

Practicing nonsexual touch can enhance your sex life in the long term. Ideas for "G-rated" touch include hugging and kissing, cuddling in bed first thing in the morning or while watching TV, putting your arm around your lover's shoulder, rubbing his or her arm or neck, and dancing cheek to cheek. Your touch should be deliberate, gentle, soft, and caring in order to have maximum effect. Think of these activities as sensual rather than sexual—they serve as reinforcements of your love for each other rather than as a sign of expectations that sexual activity will soon follow. Do not have sex in mind as your ultimate goal. Rather seek to enjoy the pleasant feelings aroused in the moment.

4. Give and receive massages.

Massage is the oldest and most intuitive form of healing. It is an integral part of Chinese medicine and several other ancient cultural traditions. It also has many health benefits. Massage stimulates the immune system, relaxes muscles, improves circulation, relieves pain, and enhances mental focus. As we discussed earlier in this section, it also stimulates the production of oxytocin. In addition, massage relieves stress, thereby facilitating a mindset conducive to sexual activity.

Massage can serve as a prelude to sex: It helps you to let go, allow yourself to be vulnerable, and therefore maximize your sexual responsiveness. It is also an excellent way to practice nonsexual, but not *nonsensual,* touch: the purpose of the massage is to stimulate your nerve endings and fully experience tactile sensation.

Here are some simple guidelines for how to *give* a massage. Although rubbing another person's body may seem intuitive, these tips can help you enjoy the experience:

1. Set up a comfortable massage environment. The room should be quiet and free from interruptions. Keep the lights low and the room temperature warm. You may want to play some calming music in the background.
2. Have your partner lie down on a sturdy, padded, flat surface that is within comfortable reach of your arms—a firm mattress or couch should do. You shouldn't have to stoop too low or stretch up too high to reach his or her body.
3. You should probably use lotion or massage oil as a lubricant to help reduce uncomfortable friction between hands and skin. However, avoid using too much lubrication—you don't want your hands to slip and slide.
4. Work rhythmically. Feel free to vary the length of your strokes, but not the timing. This will help the person you're working on to relax. You might want to try silently counting to yourself in order to keep an easy rhythm, "One . . . two . . . three . . ."
5. Use your body weight to apply pressure rather than relying on just your back and arm muscles. Lean into the massage. You'll be able to last much longer this way before getting tired. You're also less likely to suffer an injury or back pain.

6. Avoid twisting your back or otherwise straining yourself by facing the area that you are massaging.

7. Begin with large, circular strokes for a full-body warm-up. Try to direct strokes toward the heart to stimulate circulation. Apply smooth, even pressure through the palms and heels of your hands.

8. Next, work specific, small tension spots with your thumbs. Use small circular motions with firm pressure for shoulders, buttocks, and other muscular areas.

9. End the massage with long, soft, gentle strokes that cover your partner's entire body.

10. Always be attentive. Treasure your partner's body. Release tension slowly. Be careful never to gouge the skin with your fingernails, catch hair, or otherwise jar the person out of his or her restful state.

11. Imagine what it would feel like to be on the receiving end. This will help you give a more satisfying massage.

12. Encourage your partner to give you feedback. Tell him or her to let you know what feels good or when the pressure is too much.

Here are some tips for making sure that you are in optimum condition to *receive* a massage:

A. Eat a small meal beforehand. You do not want to be stuffed with food, as this will divert blood to your stomach and may make you feel uncomfortable. At the same time, you do not want to be hungry. So munch on something small and light about two hours in advance of your massage.

B. Take a few minutes to relax immediately prior to your massage. Many people find that taking a warm shower helps release muscle tension and put them in the mood. Listen to calming music, meditate, or do whatever you like to help slow your thoughts down and focus your attention on your bodily sensations.

C. Ensure that you are totally comfortable with your massage environment: No distracting noises, low lighting, warm temperature, and calming music. If you are fundamentally bothered by something in your environment, then you won't be able to fully let yourself go.

D. Breathe. Throughout the massage, inhale and exhale deeply and rhythmically. This will help you relax, focus attention on your body, and release muscle tension.

E. Communicate with your masseur or masseuse. Criticism may be distracting, but he or she will appreciate it if you offer gentle feedback about what you like and dislike. The communication need not be verbal, either—a sigh of relief or moan of pleasure can very effectively deliver the message that you are enjoying the experience.

You can exchange a quick five-minute massage with your partner or enjoy more involved, lengthy massages. Don't feel obligated to commit to a full-body massage every time, however. If you do, you are less likely to explore the sensual pleasure of massage on a regular basis. Try localized hand, foot, back, and head massages when you have less time. Also, treat yourself to a professional massage every once in a while. You will be able to fully relax—and you may pick up some great new techniques, as well.

5. Explore yourself.

Orgasm is certainly not necessary for sexual fulfillment. At the same time, learning to pleasure yourself, and even bring yourself to climax, can fundamentally improve your sexual fitness by making you responsible for your own sexuality. In general, women have more difficulty reaching orgasm than men do, but both sexes can benefit from self-exploration. Only you have the ability to let your body feel certain things; only you can allow an orgasm to happen. A partner can assist in this process but should not "make" you do anything you don't want to do.

Just like physical fitness, sexual fitness requires training. The best way to increase your sexual receptivity is to know your body, and the best way to have reliable orgasms is to practice. When you teach your body to have an orgasm, your reflexes and neural memory help it happen more easily the next time. It's like riding a bike: it takes awhile to learn, but once you get the hang of it you never forget how.

Once you become comfortable with your own body and know what enhances your desire, you are also more likely to reach orgasm during sexual activity with a partner. You can provide your lover with better feedback, tips on how to please you, and advice about what not to do. If you're interested in learning more, we recommend reading a book on the topic (e.g., Lonnie Barbach's *For Yourself* or Julia Heiman's *Becoming Orgasmic*). Take control of your own sexuality. You'll become more sexually receptive and responsive—which is only a plus for your partner, as well!

Smell

You walk by a person on the street who is wearing your lover's favorite perfume or cologne. Instantly, the scent brings to mind vivid images of lovemaking, sharing a romantic dinner, or doing a sultry dance. The perfume industry has spent billions of advertising dollars convincing us that certain scents can make us feel sexier and appear more attractive to the opposite sex. While these claims are often exaggerated, the truth is that smell plays a larger role on the stage of seduction than most people realize.

Almost every culture around the world recognizes and harnesses the power of scent. Artwork and written documents from the ancient

Chinese, Egyptian, Roman, and Aztec empires offer proof that these peoples used fragrant oils in sexual rituals from seduction to fertility rites to marriage ceremonies. Even today, lovers will scent themselves with perfumes and colognes before a big night out.

Why is olfactory sensation, the sense of smell, so important? Perhaps it is because of all the senses, smell has the most direct path to the mind. Rather than passing through some intermediary mechanism, scent molecules travel straight from the nose to the brain. Once they arrive there, smell signals are processed in the emotional center of the brain. This is why a waft of fresh baked bread or sea air can elicit such strong, immediate, and visceral responses. Although it is the simplest sense, smell can also be the most powerful one.

Scent helps determine whom we find sexy. In fact, women rate a man's smell as a crucial factor in selecting a new lover. Women are more turned on by smell than by any other sense. At the same time, they are more turned off by body odor than any single other element. Scent has a powerful impact on men, as well. In one study, men rated smell and visual cues as equally important factors in choosing a new lover.

Smell also has a direct impact on sexual arousal. Dr. Alan Hirsch of the Smell and Taste Treatment and Research Foundation in Chicago has done studies to prove it. In a series of experiments, Dr. Hirsch exposed male subjects aged eighteen to sixty-four to dozens of different odors including floral scents, perfumes, and foods. As they sniffed the odors, the doctor and his colleagues measured the degree of subjects' arousal. The researchers were surprised to discover that the smells, not of perfume, but of pumpkin pie, lavender, and black licorice caused the greatest improvements in penile blood flow among the men. In a similar experiment, women aged eighteen to forty smelled a variety of odors as researchers measured their vaginal blood flow. The women's bodies responded most to a strange and unexpected combination of licorice candy and cucumber, followed by baby powder, lavender, and pumpkin pie.

Scientists don't know why we respond to these scents the way we do. Dr. Hirsch hypothesizes that we may become aroused by food odors because our ancestors used to congregate and meet their mates around the fire at mealtimes. Or the explanation could be more straightforward: Smells relax us and remind us of pleasurable experiences. For example, perhaps the scent of baby powder makes women feel wistful. For both men and women, the smell of pumpkin pie may conjure up images of warm, happy times with family during the holidays.

Aside from the naturally occurring food smells that we've just discussed, another obvious way to make use of your sense of smell is to wear manufactured scents. As a society, we literally buy into the idea that perfumes, colognes, powders, body sprays, and the like can make us feel sexier and even seem more attractive to others: we spend billions of dollars a year on these products. While no clinical evidence exists regarding the actual effect of perfumes on sexual arousal, it is true that certain scents are associated with specific meanings. Your choice of perfume or cologne can send clear messages about yourself to others (see chart on next page).

Regardless of the reasons, we know that scents work to enhance sexual fitness. There are many ways for you to experiment with this powerful and underutilized sense: Cook the foods listed above; fill your home with scented candles, potpourris, and incense; try wearing different perfumes and colognes; massage each other with scented oils. Whatever you do, use your imagination.

Aromatherapy

Aromatherapy, which involves using the natural, concentrated oils (known as essential oils) of plants for therapeutic purposes, is another way to put your sense of smell to work for you. Although it is now considered "alternative" medicine, the practice of using scents to heal dates back to ancient Egypt, more than 5,000 years ago.

PERFUMES AND COLOGNES: CHOOSING A SCENT

SCENT	WHERE THE SCENT COMES FROM	WHAT THE SCENT IMPLIES
Herb, plant	Eucalyptus, marjoram, mint, rosemary, camphor, lavender, etc.	Clean, fresh, outdoorsy, adventuresome
Musk	Glandular secretion of musk deer, civet cat, and beavers Found in small intestines of sperm whale	Sensuous, sexual, seductive
Flower	Rose, narcissus, jasmine, violet, lily, hyacinth, etc.	Feminine, fertile, youthful
Citrus fruit	Orange, lemon, and lime	Lively, clean, professional
Earth	Roots, soil, moss, and other plants	Warm, mellow, natural
Spice	Cloves, cinnamon, cassia, bay laurel, etc.	Mysterious, exotic, seductive

According to aromatherapists and popular tradition, the power of scent may be harnessed to potentially help address sexual concerns. Aromatherapy practitioners try to elevate desire by performing a massage with rose, jasmine, ylang ylang, clary sage, or sandalwood. Bathing in sandalwood or being massaged with jasmine, neroli (orange blossom), and clary sage, they claim, can diminish erectile dysfunction (ED). Rose essence is used to help people who are sterile or infertile. For menopause, practitioners recommend sage for depression and hot flashes, as well as licorice, rose, and jasmine. For PMS, they suggest a massage with geranium and rosemary oil. Jasmine, lavender, and sandalwood can soothe anxiety and induce a calm, relaxed state of mind. The essential oils are never taken internally, but rather applied to the skin through massage or bathing in scented water, or simply inhaled through diffusion.

You can experiment with aromatherapy without the aid of a professional. There are many ways to enjoy the potentially arousing and healing effects of scent. Involve your partner in an activity, or simply treat yourself to some special time alone—what you learn can benefit your own state of mind as well as your next experience as a couple. Make your aromatherapy practices ritualistic by ensuring that you have plenty of time as well as a calm environment in which to relax and inhale the scents surrounding you. Never ingest aromatherapy oil, and use only a small amount of the concentrated essential oil in any of the combinations listed below.

Here are a few ideas for ways to "aromatherapize" yourself:

- Burn a scented candle.
- Use an aromatherapy diffuser, a small instrument available at many alternative health and beauty stores, to disperse the scent of essential oils.
- Spray a combination of essential oil and water onto your skin and wear it as a perfume. Don't use very much, however, as these scents can quickly become overwhelming.
- Add a drop or two of essential oil or bath oil to hot water and bathe in it.
- Dab some essential oil on a piece of cloth and leave it in your closet or drawer to subtly scent your clothes and lingerie.
- Mix a small amount of essential oil with regular body oil for massage. Be careful to keep this scented oil from direct contact with your genitals, and never use it as a lubricant.

Pheromones

For animals, the nose is more valuable than the eyes, ears, or any other sensory organ. That's because animals rely primarily on pheromones to communicate. Pheromones are odorless, tasteless chemical signals secreted by one animal and picked up by other members of its species. The pheromone then elicits an automatic, uncontrolled behavioral response from the animal that senses it. In this way, pheromones serve to deliver messages from one member of a species to another. For example, pheromones help bees tell other bees how to navigate their way to food. When dogs and wolves urinate to mark their territory, it is pheromones that communicate the "I was here" message to others of the breed.

FITNESS FACT

Pheromones are chemicals secreted by animals that help them to communicate with other members of their species. Even though the sense organ that detects pheromones, the vomeronasal organ (VNO), is located in the nose, pheromones are not smells nor are they processed in the same manner as are smells.

The impact of pheromones on human behavior is not well understood. It is clear that these chemicals do not govern us in the powerful way that they control animals. Yet pheromones might have some subtle, subconscious effects on our responses to others, as well as our sociability and general mood. So far, we don't have a lot of research to go on. This is due in large part to the fact that, until recently, scientists did not think that humans had the necessary equipment to sense pheromones. Only in 1993 did they discover the existence of the vomeronasal organ, or VNO, in adults.

The VNO consists of two tiny holes located inside the nose. This organ, although housed inside the nose and sharing the same physical structure as the olfactory organs, acts completely independently from scent. Without the VNO, chemical communication via pheromones would be impossible.

If pheromones are detected by the VNO, where are they produced? They appear to be released by glands located in the underarms, genital area, and other parts of the body. The close proximity of these glands to sweat glands indicates that pheromones can be dispersed and transferred from person to person via sweat, and therefore inhaled easily, especially during sex.

The strongest evidence for the power of human pheromones comes from studies of the female reproductive cycle. Psychologist Martha McClintock of the University of Chicago first noticed years ago that women who lived together in college dormitories often ended up with synchronized menstrual cycles. The more time they spent together, the more likely that the onset of their cycles would match.

This finding intrigued McClintock, so she decided to try an experiment. She exposed a group of women to other women's sweat. The study went like this: A group of women wore pads under their arms for two days. Then the sweat was collected from the pads and swabbed under the trial subjects' noses. McClintock found that within months the trial women's cycles would synchronize with the menstrual cycles of the women whose sweat they smelled—even though the women themselves had no physical contact with one another. She believes that the effect must, therefore, have been created by pheromones.

Other studies show that women who have sex with men at least once a week have more regular menstrual cycles and higher estrogen levels than do women who are not having sex. Scientists believe that this enhanced fertility in copulating women is generated by pheromones because it does not occur through masturbation alone, but only after spending a significant amount of time with a male partner.

In general, it seems that pheromones do indeed have some impact on human sexual behavior. The most likely scenario is that pheromones send unconscious messages that influence our "gut feelings" about others. For example, many people believe that pheromones determine who we are attracted to right away. Then, as we get to know people better, other factors such as personality and social status assume greater importance. Further scientific research is needed to define the specific role of human pheromones on sexual arousal and response.

Taste

Food and sex: They share an intimate bond, as they each give us life. They are also two of the greatest sensual pleasures, and are often enjoyed together. Edibles can enhance and enrich the sexual experience in several different ways.

Food has a relationship with sex that goes beyond its strict nutritional value. Food can play an instrumental role in sexual seduction, arousal, and the act of sex itself. Think, for example, of how sensual eating can be. Have you ever watched a woman seductively pull a cherry off its stem and let its juices run down her chin? Or gazed in lust as a man slowly savors his martini, tongue first? You can enjoy a sensuous meal—in the form of a romantic dinner at a restaurant, a delicious home-cooked meal, or a simple picnic outdoors—as a precursor to sexual activity. You can also actually bring foods into the bedroom. Try feeding each other or, if you're feeling more playful and daring, eating off of one another.

Different foods provide for different stimulating sexual adventures. The Japanese consider sushi highly sensual. In the United States, chocolate and oysters are traditionally viewed as erotic. Fruits—including apples, pears, figs, and grapes—serve as sexual symbols in literature that spans cultures and centuries, from the Bible's *Song of Solomon* to the Indian *Kama Sutra* to modern-day erotica. This tremendous breadth of opinion just goes to show that fun with food all depends upon your personal taste and creativity. So pick up a piece of chocolate or a juicy cherry—it's up to you!

Aside from the seductive powers of food, taste can contribute directly to sexual pleasure. As we discussed in the section on smell, scientific research shows that certain scents directly stimulate sexual excitement. Since taste is 90 percent smell, it is likely that eating foods with those scents affects sexual arousal as much as—if not more than—does smelling them alone. Think of some of the most potent scents listed earlier, such as pumpkin pie and lavender. If smelling pumpkin pie causes genital blood flow to increase, shouldn't eating the pie have a similar effect? You may want to seduce your lover by cooking or going out for a romantic dinner. Perhaps at least one way to a person's heart is, after all, through the stomach.

Also, there is another way to put your sense of taste to work for your sexual pleasure. In popular culture, mints are legendary for enhancing oral sex. The story goes that if you chew on a mint just prior to giving your partner oral sex, you'll drive him or her to new levels of sexual ecstasy. Actually, there seems to be a physiological explanation for this phenomenon. Peppermint causes mild irritation to the skin. This creates a warm, pleasant tingling sensation and serves to increase surface blood flow to the region, making the mind more attuned to what is going on. As a result, your mint may improve your partner's performance as well as stimulating his or her awareness of and sensation in the genital region. So the next time you're ready to pleasure your lover, try munching on a mint or taking a swig of crème de menthe before you begin.

Sound

What could be more important for setting a romantic mood than music? It's hard to imagine a candlelit dinner for two without the elegant accompaniment of guitar music or love songs playing in the background. And yet many of us forget to harness the power of music in our daily lives. You can easily stimulate your libido by controlling the sounds that surround you.

A growing body of research suggests that sound vibrations cause the brain to produce alpha waves. Alpha waves, which can be detected by EEGs (electroencephalograms), indicate a relaxed state of mind. Some scientists believe that an alpha state promotes the healing process, generates feelings of well-being, and also enhances mental acuity, intuition, and creativity. As a result, sound vibration therapy is increasingly recognized as a practical means to relieve stress, improve concentration, induce deeper and more restful sleep, and boost energy levels. Some researchers believe that listening to music may even increase intelligence, the so-called "Mozart effect."

In terms of sexual fitness, music can improve your mood, help you de-stress, stimulate your mind, soothe your body, and otherwise prepare you for sexual activity after a long day spent at work or taking care of the kids. Music is a well-established tool for altering people's moods. Psychologists often play music to make their subjects feel a certain way. For example, classical music is frequently used in experiments to induce feelings of elation, although tribal or repetitious music might prove more stimulating in sexual situations.

Music may have a direct impact on sexual arousal, as well. In a clinical trial conducted at Boston University, when men listened to music that induced a negative mood they showed decreased penile tumescence (the scientific term for how hard an erection gets) relative to the silent control condition. When they listened to positive mood music, on the other hand, they experienced greater penile tumescence and reported that they were more aroused than when not listening to music. This is hardly surprising, as music can help create an erotic environment.

There are many different musical genres to choose from including classical, New Age, soft rock, ambient, tribal rhythms, and even more esoteric forms like Japanese drums or Gregorian chants. Aside from music, sounds from nature such as that of a babbling brook, rainfall, or pounding surf can also serve as an excellent backdrop for sex. Some people find listening to the underwater songs of whales incredibly erotic!

While no one genre is more conducive to sexual enjoyment than any other, it is critical that the music put you in a mood that makes you feel receptive to sex. How a specific piece of music affects you depends on your perception of it. If the sounds make you feel sexy, sensuous, or aroused, then they work for you, and that's what matters.

Spend time with your partner listening to tunes and picking out your favorite sexual accompaniments. Then don't forget to actually put the music on when you're ready for a romantic tryst. In a short period of time, playing certain songs can act as a sexual cue for you and your partner; a sign that pleasure is soon to come. Like the music "Bolero" in the movie *Ten*, you can develop themes for yourself and your lover. These songs will have an inherent meaning for the two of you. Just hearing a few notes can titillate you and start you down a path of sexual intimacy that you may not have been in the mood for earlier.

Another option is to embrace the sensual beauty of silence so that you can hear the sounds of each other's ecstasy. Listen to your breathing, moans and groans, sighs and screams. Feel free to make as much noise as you like. Many people find the natural, uncontrolled sounds that we tend to make during sex highly arousing. In addition, these sounds serve as a form of nonverbal communication between you and your lover, signaling when you are reaching the heights of ecstasy. After listening to each other, you may find that your own music is your favorite music of all.

Finally, you can enhance the sexual experience by talking to each other. During sexual activity, verbally encourage your lover. When your partner does something particularly enjoyable, let him or her know. If something does not feel good to you, simply demonstrate an alternative or divert the action. Teach each other what you find most pleasing. Gently tell your lover your dislikes at another time: criticism has no place in eroticism, so you should discuss these issues outside of the sexual context.

Some people enjoy erotic talk during lovemaking. Whisper positive words of approval or love into your partner's ear. Compliment each other on how sexy you look or feel. Or, if you're in the mood for play and your lover agrees to it in advance, say something raunchy. A majority of men and women report that they enjoy "dirty talk." Experiment to find out what tone of voice, words, phrases, or messages most turn your lover on. Think of your vocal cords as yet another bodily instrument of sexual pleasure.

Sight

You see someone whom you consider sexy walking down the street. What happens? You become subtly aware of your body. You feel flushed and your heart races. You may even start to feel sexually aroused.

Humans differ from most other animals in that our eyes are organs of erotic stimulation. We can become sexually aroused by visual stimuli alone. Think of the traditional tools used for sexual arousal: we often take pleasure from looking at sexy pictures and from reading literature filled with erotic visual imagery.

Both men and women can benefit by using their sense of sight to enhance sexual pleasure. Aside from looking at suggestive pictures in a magazine or watching a sexy movie, reading a romance novel or erotica, here are a few ideas for how to make use of this important tool.

Color and Light

What we see in our surroundings influences our desire for sex. You can change how things appear and even how you feel by playing with different lighting schemes. Have you ever noticed that romantic dinners are often held by candlelight and that Hollywood seduction scenes frequently occur in front of a burning fire? This is probably due to the fact that fire and candles provide the most flattering light. Perhaps because of fire's primal nature, it seems to ensure the right mood for sex. It can make us feel warm, happy, and less inhibited.

Soft lighting is sexy, so don't save it for special occasions. Make use of fires in the fireplace, candles, low-powered lightbulbs with warm, pink tones or dimmer switches, indirect lighting and shadows to help create an atmosphere of love in your home all the time. The moon also offers a light that is soft and subtle, romantic and erotic. Take advantage of moonlight by spending time outside—or at least near a window—with your lover when the weather cooperates.

Colors may also play a role in sexual desire by having an impact on your mood. Use the chart below to help you determine how you might be able to enhance your sexual desire by changing the color scheme of your bedroom. For example, if you often find yourself too fatigued for sexual activity, add some red. If you are anxious and high-strung, your bedroom should help you relax. Make green, purple, and blue the dominant colors. Yellow is best if you are often sad and need an emotional pickup to feel sexy. You might also experiment with var-

HOW COLORS INFLUENCE SEXUAL AROUSAL	
Red	Arouses and stimulates
Blue	Relaxes and calms
Yellow	Revitalizes and cheers
Green	Soothes and comforts
Purple	Inspires and cools

ious combinations of colors. And don't just think about the paint on your walls—you can also change the colors of your sheets, pillows, curtains, pictures, and even your bedclothes.

Objects of Desire

In addition to color, think about the actual objects and items that you want to have around you while making love. When couples go in for counseling, one of the first questions many sex therapists will ask is "How is your bedroom set up?" Although this may seem like a ridiculous and irrelevant topic, it is actually quite important to maintaining optimum sexual fitness. You see, people tend to clutter their bedrooms with all sorts of objects that have nothing to do with sleep or sex: TVs, piles of dirty laundry, exercise gear, even home office equipment. The problem arises when people use their bedrooms more for unfinished work of all kinds than for pleasure. Instead of being a safe haven, a place the couple views as comfortable, peaceful, and erotic, the bedroom becomes just another room in the house—a place associated with stress, arguments, and work.

> **FITNESS FACT**
>
> **Your bedroom should be a sacred place where only sex and sleeping occur.**

In order to prevent this problem from arising, you should remove all distractions from the bedroom. If possible, move the TV, exercise equipment, and home office to other rooms of the house, or at least behind closet doors or screens. These objects distract your brain with nonsexual thoughts, rather than allowing you to pay full attention to sexual stimulation and relaxation. If you can't clear out your bedroom, then at least put a curtain or room divider between your bed and the part of the room that you use for other activities.

Now you can think about turning this space into a den of sensual pleasures by enhancing it with positive visual cues, such as pillows and blankets, fresh flowers and plants, and—don't forget—soft lighting. Try to provide yourself with a bedroom atmosphere that you and your lover enjoy and find sexually arousing. Experiment with different environmental elements to determine which please you the most. Redecorating may be as simple as stringing lights across the wall or at the base of the bed, buying some extra-soft cushions, putting your mattress on the floor, or adding drapes over your bed. Make yourself a true love nest. It's worth the money and the effort.

Eye Contact

As the saying goes, "The eyes are the windows to the soul." Eye contact is a powerful way to connect with other people. Yet we often either avoid this intimacy, forget about it, or feel too self-conscious to make eye contact with our lovers. In our society, we're encouraged to keep our eyes closed and the lights off—to have sex, literally and figuratively, in the dark. As a result of these behaviors, we may miss out on the deep sexual connection that can be made through intense eye contact. Also, many people may feel shy about allowing their partners to see their bodies during lovemaking. The truth is that lovers are hardly ever critical, but rather have an appreciation for their partners' bodies: It is usually a large part of their arousal. Maximal stimulation and inner connection can occur with "eyes open" sex.

Try this exercise to intensify your lovemaking and reach new levels of intimacy with your partner. Have some soft, gentle lighting; or, if you are already accustomed to it, leave the lights on. Begin by making eye contact with your partner for a few minutes during foreplay. Take your time. When you get bolder, establish eye contact while you are in the process of genital stimulation or even sexual intercourse itself. Gradually work yourselves up to more and more extended periods of eye contact. Eventually, you may be able to go through an entire sexual session without looking away from your lover's eyes. This can be an incredibly rewarding experience.

Visualization

Another way you can potentially enhance your sexual abilities or comfort level is to practice visualization techniques. For years, athletes have been trained to imagine a perfect performance. Visualization is now a well-publicized and accepted technique used in sex therapy. After all, if visualization helps athletes improve their mental and physical fitness, why not use it to improve sexual fitness?

Visualizing sexual events has several potential benefits. You can use it to help you focus better: by practicing visualization techniques, you can learn to be more present in your body and experience arousal more fully. You may also use visualization to aid in relaxation: imagining pleasurable activities can put you in the mood for sex. Finally, visualization can be helpful if you feel awkward, uncomfortable, or insecure in any way about sexual activity. Sex therapists sometimes encourage patients who have difficulty reaching orgasm to visualize as they are approaching the finale of the sex act. Doing so keeps them centered on the pleasure they are feeling rather than on distracting thoughts. The key to visualization is that there are no performance expectations—just your own imagination. It's like practicing without anyone there to watch or judge you.

Begin by lying down in a comfortable, quiet place where you'll be assured no interruptions. Close your eyes and breathe deeply. Once you feel yourself relax, you can start the visualization process. Picture yourself looking sexy, then conjure up the image of your partner or an attractive imaginary lover. Now imagine yourself performing each and every action that you would want to take in this situation, from lightly touching your lover's skin with your hand, to a gentle kiss, to reaching your sexual peak.

The key to visualization success is focusing on the details. Do not rush through this process. Concentrate on making the events actually unfold in your mind's eye. Imagine every sensation: what you feel like, what you see, what you smell, what you hear. Be creative and confident.

Allow yourself to imagine all the wonderful things you would like to do with your loved one without fear of failure and without hesitation. Remember, there is no risk!

Repeat the exercise as often as you like. It will become easier every time. When the vision is clearly ingrained in your mind, experiencing the scenarios you've imagined will become that much easier.

Tantric Sex

We've seen what each and every one of our senses can do to enhance sexual fitness. One sexual philosophy that makes optimal use of sensual stimulation is Tantra. You may have heard of it—there's quite a buzz these days about Tantric sex. This ancient practice, which has been taught for thousands of years in the East, has recently caught on in the West. Seminars, books, videos, and experts on the topic multiply by the day. Many people who participate in Tantric rituals claim that they revitalize their sex lives.

What is Tantra? Tantra is about fully exploring the senses in order to maximize pleasure. The techniques involve focusing attention on breathing, kissing, touching, and deeply experiencing every sensation. This Indian tradition seeks to help people develop themselves spiritually through sexual expression. In Sanskrit, Tantra means "to weave" or "to integrate." Tantric ritual offers a way of achieving deeper sexual connections with others. It involves practicing exercises such as sustained eye contact, massage, erotic kissing, synchronized breathing, and advanced lovemaking techniques. It also encourages you to move slowly. The goal of Tantra is not orgasm or improved performance, but rather to enhance your awareness of pleasure and how you relate as a couple.

Here is a quick summary of five Tantric sex exercises that you can try. If you're interested in finding out more, you may want to take a class or purchase a book. This is only a brief outline of a few techniques—certainly not enough to help you learn the intricacies of Tantra.

1. Establish a shared ritual.

Spend time with your partner creating a ritual that makes the sexual act sacred. This ritual can involve words or objects or both—it's only important the ritual have meaning for you. Some examples of rituals include bathing each other, giving each other massages, or exchanging gifts. Practice your ritual prior to engaging in Tantric sex.

2. Perform synchronized breathing.

Lie together on a bed touching each other. Allow yourselves to breathe in perfect harmony. Doing so will help you get rid of distracting thoughts and focus only on the other person. If you feel yourself struggling to stay in synch, relax and let go. As long as you concentrate, the process of coordinating your breathing patterns should come naturally.

3. Engage in sustained eye contact.

While you are lying together, stare deeply into your partner's eyes. Never remove your gaze. You should feel an intense connection to each other. This activity may feel awkward at first as, but you will quickly grow accustomed to it. There is no better way to ensure intimacy during sex than through eye contact.

4. Practice motionless intercourse.

During the sexual peak of intercourse, but before orgasm, stop moving. Hold still for several minutes. Concentrate on the sensations that you experience in those moments. The stillness, in stark contrast to the constant motion of typical intercourse, will give you time to reflect on your intimate union with your partner. As you become more advanced, remain motionless for longer periods of time.

5. Have sex without orgasm.

This exercise will help shift your focus during sex from orgasm to the sensual experience. By practicing sexual activity without orgasm, you will realize the full range of sexual pleasure available to you. Let go. Stop worrying about when you will climax. Instead, concentrate completely on what you are feeling in the moment.

Sensual stimulation can motivate you to participate in sexual activity when you're not in the mood by arousing your desire and making you feel sexy. It can help you relax, so that your mind slows down and lets go of its concerns. It can give you the opportunity to experience physical enjoyment in ways that don't always lead to sexual activity, so that you feel safe and comfortable with intimacy. It can assist you in discovering your likes and dislikes, and empower you to take control of your own sexual pleasure. And it can just be plain fun!

Now that you've learned the benefits of fully employing all your senses, you can begin to experiment. You'll find simple and, we hope, enjoyable sensual stimulation exercises to try throughout the Sexual Fitness Program. Much of the program involves intense effort on your part in terms of eating a healthy diet; cutting back on alcohol, cigarettes, and other substances; getting plenty of exercise and sleep; and relieving stress. So it's especially important that you take the time to engage in these sensual stimulation activities, either alone or with a partner. They will allow you to enjoy your sexuality in a playful way at the same time that you're enhancing your sexual fitness. What could be better?

Try not to rely solely on the suggestions offered here. You may have heard the saying "The mind is the most powerful sexual organ there is." Go beyond the recommendations provided in the book and explore your own imagination. You are limited only by your own reservations and self-imposed boundaries. Challenge yourself to reach a whole new dimension of sensuality.

Creativity is an amazing gift. Put it to work for you.

5

Exercise

When you make a commitment to better sexuality, you make a commitment to better health. That's the beauty of sexual fitness—what's good for your sexual health is good for your overall wellness. Being physically active is the most straightforward way for you to take control of both these vital aspects of your life. Physical fitness and sexual fitness are inextricably linked. By engaging in regular physical activity—whether in the form of jogging, biking, swimming, or doing t'ai chi—you have the power to make yourself feel more sexual and assert a long-lasting positive impact on your overall wellness.

Physical activity is a major priority in achieving sexual fitness because sexual performance and pleasure depend on a healthy heart and low cholesterol levels, ensuring adequate blood flow to the genitals and other regions of the body. When you're active, you increase your lean body mass and make your body a more efficient fat-burning machine, which makes it easier to maintain an appropriate weight (which we will also discuss in this chapter). Exercise also builds endurance, flexibility, muscle strength, and bone density. And, most important, it has an impact on your sex life by enhancing your self-esteem and increasing your physical stamina. Over time, with regular physical activity, your body will change in ways that facilitate better sex.

There is simply no question that exercising will enhance your sex life. Many research studies as well as real-life observations demonstrate that, regardless of age, men and women who are physically active enjoy greater levels of sexual activity and pleasure than do their nonactive cohorts. In a clinical trial of sedentary but healthy middle-aged men, the group that exercised the most experienced the most significant improvements in cardiovascular and sexual fitness. After nine months of regular workouts, these men engaged in more frequent sexual activity, had fewer problems with erectile dysfunction (ED), and reported a higher percentage of satisfying orgasms.

Physical activity works in three primary ways to physiologically enhance sexual function. First, it has a direct impact on your cardiovascular health. When you consume a nutritionally poor diet and do not exercise, cholesterol collects inside your artery walls, narrowing these delicate vessels. As a result, an adequate amount of blood cannot reach the genitalia. Erections in men and arousal in women often suffer. In fact, arteriosclerosis (narrowing of the arteries from cholesterol and fat deposits) is one of the primary causes of sexual dysfunction.

Physical activity gets your metabolism pumping, which helps reduce cholesterol levels. The combination of eating a healthy diet and exercising regularly will significantly lower levels of "bad" LDL cholesterol while increasing or maintaining levels of "good" HDL cholesterol. This process keeps your arteries clear so that blood can flow freely to the genitals and other areas of the body. Therefore, when physically fit, men are less likely to experience ED and women are more likely to enjoy full genital arousal and sexual satisfaction.

Second, exercise serves to boost production of key sex hormones. Several studies have shown that testosterone levels rise just after short periods of intense exercise. According to one Canadian clinical trial, men's testosterone levels increased during exercise, peaked twenty to thirty minutes after the session, and then declined. A similar effect was observed in a trial involving women, with testosterone levels significantly higher fifteen to thirty minutes after physical activity. Over the long term, men and women who regularly work out have higher overall levels of testosterone than do nonactive people, as well. This may translate into a more active and satisfying sex life.

Testosterone production is a particularly critical issue for people over fifty. Recall from chapter 3: *Medications* that testosterone levels fall in both men and women with age. When testosterone levels are abnormally low, desire for sexual activity and response to sexual stimuli can seriously decline. Exercise, in combination with a balanced diet, can act as a natural form of testosterone replacement therapy (TRT), helping the body to compensate for this loss.

Estrogen levels in women can also be raised by exercise. The dramatic drop in estrogen that occurs with menopause can create many unpleasant side effects. Studies show that, for a majority of women, exercising regularly effectively reduces hot flashes, sweating, and mood swings caused by menopause. Women suffering from these problems should regard exercise and a proper diet as their first line of defense against the menopausal loss of estrogen.

Third, exercise has a positive impact on overall health and wellness by increasing physical energy and stamina, partly by reducing weight and body fat, and partly by improving cardiovascular function. This may explain why people who are physically fit claim that they can last longer—they simply don't tire out as easily. And let's not forget that exercise builds flexibility and strength, which can both be of real value.

Physical activity has numerous benefits from a psychological perspective, as well. Most of us are probably familiar with the feel-good sensation that comes from a satisfying workout. Exercise boosts the level of endorphins, the chemicals in the brain that are responsible for generating a warm, happy feeling. This rise in endorphin levels may account for the so-called "runner's high." Exercise also relieves anxiety and improves mood, as is evident in the case of Albert.

FITNESS FACT

Exercise causes the brain to release endorphins, or pleasure signals—the same chemicals released when we fall in love.

Albert has discovered that exercise has a direct impact on his sex drive. He is a VP at a high-tech company. At forty-two, he is in generally good health. He has always enjoyed a strong libido and considers himself a very sexual man. But his job can be overwhelmingly demanding and stressful at times.

In the past few years, as his responsibilities at work grew, Albert began to feel his sexual appetite seriously decline. He discovered that he only had the energy to engage in sexual activity on the weekends. The rest of the time, he complained, he just wanted to go home and sleep. He felt frustrated and also concerned about his health.

Albert decided to take control of the situation. He made his health—with the motivation to get back to his old sexual self—a priority. He started making the time to run regularly. After just one month, he could already feel the difference. "Exercise changes everything for me," says Albert. "It's transforming."

He has continued to work out at least four times a week and now has more energy and feels less anxious about his job and his lifestyle. What's more, he has experienced a noticeable boost to his sex drive. Therefore, regardless of how busy he gets, Albert is committed to keeping up with his exercise regimen.

In older men and women, the relationship between physical activity and sexuality is particularly significant. As discussed in previous chapters, our cardiovascular health, hormone production, and overall energy levels naturally tend to decline as we age. However, these changes are not inevitable. Exercise can help keep you in excellent cardiovascular condition and also boost your hormone and energy levels. A Stanford University survey of men and women over fifty concluded that self-rated sexual satisfaction and physical fitness were highly correlated, even in the seventy-plus age group.

As you can see, physical fitness is a powerful, effective way to achieve sexual fitness. Working out will enhance many crucial aspects of your sexual well-being, both psychologically and physiologically.

Tips for Getting Going

For many of us, maintaining even a mild level of physical activity can be a challenge. You may have been meaning to exercise for ages, but just never get around to it. Or perhaps you work out from time to time but have trouble sticking to a routine. Well, now you have your incentive: Exercise will improve your sex life. You can gain control of your cardiovascular, physical, and sexual fitness by making this critical change. You have the power to make a tremendous difference in how you feel, your energy levels, as well as your libido and sexual performance. It's all up to you. You have the motivation, you have the ability, and you have the strength. Get going today!

Here are some tips for how to get started with an exercise program and stick to it:

1. Pick activities that you enjoy.

   Don't force yourself to run if you hate running, because you won't keep it up. You can walk, swim, bicycle, do aerobics, or practice yoga. You can even learn to box, golf, ballroom-dance, or bowl. The specific activities you choose matter far less than the fact that you like them.

2. Make sure that exercising is convenient.

The activities you select should be easy for you to do. Don't choose swimming as your form of exercise if it takes an hourlong special trip to get to the pool. Try to work out near either your home or office. Make sure that you have options for physical activities whether it's raining, snowing, or a bright sunny day.

3. Don't let yourself get bored.

Experiment with new activities. For example, if you like ice skating, try in-line skating. Also, rather than taking the same class or doing the same workout every day of the week, rotate your schedule. Swim one day, then do aerobics the next. Do a long-distance run for one workout, and then do sprints for the next. By keeping yourself entertained, you are more likely to stay motivated.

4. Work out with a buddy.

Exercise buddies will help motivate you and prevent you from coming up with excuses for not working out. You can motivate your buddy, too. You're a lot less likely to skip a walk around the park or trip to the gym if you know that your friend is counting on you, and vice versa. Some people enjoy working out with their spouses. Exercising together gives couples time to enjoy each other in the midst of their busy lives—and you may even end up in the bedroom for a different kind of workout!

5. Take classes or join an activity group.

A trained instructor will be able to help address your specific needs, give you advice on how to stay fit, and keep you motivated. Also, being part of a group will ensure that you have regularly scheduled activities to attend, so you'll be less likely to skip your day's workout. Aside from classes at a gym, many communities have walking groups, running clubs, soccer or basketball teams, and other adult exercise groups that you can join free of charge.

6. Make time to stretch.

Start your workouts with a warm-up: Get your muscles heated up with about five minutes of physical activity, then stretch.

Stretch again for at least five minutes at the end of your workout. Stretching will reduce your risk of injury, prevent you from getting sore, and make you more flexible.

7. Begin today; no excuses.

Don't tell yourself, "I'll start next week because I have a big project due on Friday" or "I just need to get over this little cold." As soon as you check with your physician to make sure that it's okay, get started with your new exercise routine. Put on a pair of tennis shoes and take a walk around the house. Join a gym. Walk up a flight of stairs. You may only do ten minutes of physical activity, but you will have taken the first critical step—both physically and mentally. Start today!

8. Start slowly.

Don't push yourself too hard, especially at first. You've got to give your body time to get used to the idea of exercise and you certainly don't want to begin by injuring yourself. So do what you can, but don't overdo it. You'll know when you're ready for more. Also, be sure to allow yourself a day of rest after a particularly strenuous workout. You can go for a walk or work in the garden every day of the week, but for more serious physical activity it's best to give your body a chance to recover.

9. Listen to your body.

If you have a sore knee, don't keep pushing yourself to walk harder and faster. Pay attention to your aches and pains. You do not want a mild irritation to become a serious injury, which could potentially slow you down for months. So when your body says "Stop!"—do it. Then make an appointment to see your physician and figure out how you can fix the problem before it gets worse.

10. Set goals.

Make weekly goals for yourself—think about what you will achieve and write it down. A goal can be as simple as "I'm going to go to the gym four times this week." Once you get more advanced, you can set yourself more complex goals, such as "I'm going to take five minutes off my running time." If you really want to make sure that you'll stick to your goals, share them with another person. You'll be less likely to "cheat" if you do.

11. Reward yourself.

You shouldn't treat yourself to an ice-cream sundae after every workout, but there are other ways for you to motivate yourself with simple rewards. You might buy yourself a new pair of workout clothes or training shoes after completing a month of regular exercise, throw a party to celebrate three months of commitment to physical activity, or simply reward yourself by taking a long look at yourself in the mirror and congratulating yourself on your achievement. You deserve it!

Types of Exercise

Depending on your current level of physical fitness, your sexual fitness goal is most likely to gradually work your way up to at least thirty minutes of exercise, three to four times a week. Now that you know the level of physical activity that you should target and are ready to get started, the next question is: What type of exercise should you choose to do? As a general rule, you should pick whatever form of physical activity you enjoy the most, whatever will keep you motivated. There are plenty of options even for the exercise hater, and we'll discuss just a few of them in this section. We'll also reveal if certain types of exercise might have the potential to damage your sexual abilities.

If you, like many Americans, are not already involved in a regular exercise program, here are some ideas for what to do. Clinical trials have demonstrated that regularly engaging in moderate-intensity exercise reduces your risk of heart disease just as effectively as high-intensity exercise does. The goal is simply to get moving, increase your heart rate, boost your metabolism, and burn some calories. You can do it!

Exercise

Walking is an excellent way for you to get a regular dose of physical activity. Here are just a few of its benefits:

- You can do it anywhere at any time, outside (on the streets, at a park) or inside (on a treadmill, around your house, in a shopping mall).
- It doesn't require any equipment other than a pair of walking shoes.
- You don't have to learn any new skills.
- You don't need to have any special abilities, such as hand-eye coordination.
- You can do it alone or with a friend, in silence or listening to music.
- It has a low risk of injury.
- It's good for your heart and your health.

Research shows that walking effectively controls hypertension and lowers your risk of heart disease. A study published in *Circulation*, the journal of the American Heart Association, examined the effects of walking on men aged seventy-one to ninety-three. Results showed that taking daily walks, regardless of speed, substantially reduced the men's risk of heart disease. The farther the men walked, the more their heart disease risk fell: a 15 percent decrease for every half mile covered. In a similar study of middle-aged women, walking regularly (three or more hours per week) and at a brisk pace significantly reduced the incidence of heart disease.

There are many other types of physical activity besides walking, such as yoga, water aerobics, tennis, dancing, golf, and swimming. Some people enjoy an ancient Chinese form of exercise called t'ai chi. T'ai chi, which involves slow, graceful movements and deep breathing, is commonly practiced in China to this day. It has recently been gaining popularity in the United States as an especially appealing option for older people, who are prone to injury, as it focuses on controlled muscle movements rather than heavy impact and sweat. In a clinical trial, a group of sedentary adults over age sixty did t'ai chi four days a week, thirty minutes per day. They experienced a reduction in blood pressure just as significant as that of a group participating in an equal amount of aerobic exercise. They also showed improvements in balance.

Recent scientific evidence indicates that you don't have to engage in structured, organized sports such as aerobics, basketball, or tennis in order to reap the benefits of physical activity. Even everyday activities that require exertion—or "lifestyle activities," as they've come to be known—such as walking up the stairs, gardening, housecleaning, and raking the leaves, can be effective forms of exercise.

Two studies published by the *Journal of the American Medical Association* reveal that "lifestyle activity" may offer similar benefits to structured aerobic exercise. One of the studies involved obese middle-aged women. After sixteen weeks, the women in the lifestyle group (thirty minutes physical activity per day) had lost just as much weight as the aerobic exercise group (three forty-five-minute step classes per week), and their cholesterol levels were significantly reduced. What's more, participants who did lifestyle exercise were more likely to stick to their exercise regimen over time. The other trial involved previously sedentary men and women aged thirty-five to sixty. After two years, those in the lifestyle group demonstrated similar improvements in activity level, cardiorespiratory fitness, and blood pressure to the structured-activity group (aerobic activity for twenty to sixty minutes at least three times per week).

Lifestyle exercise is a great way to get started on a program of regular physical activity. It is particularly advantageous for people who don't have the time for structured activities, dislike vigorous exercise, or lack access to facilities and equipment (especially during poor weather). It involves doing your "exercise" as you go, like parking at the far end of the parking lot so that you have to walk the quarter mile to your office building or walking around the house during TV commercials, or shoveling snow. It's easy to do, fits into any lifestyle, and is beneficial to your health. There's simply no excuse not to give it a try!

Finding a Balance

We've clearly seen how exercise can enhance sexual fitness. The chart below guides you through the various levels of exercise, from mild to moderate to intense, so that you can find the appropriate level for you. Most people should strive to achieve a moderate level of exercise. Activities that will help you attain this goal include brisk walking or jogging, weight training, aerobics classes, swimming, cycling, and many team sports.

EXERCISE GUIDE

ACTIVITY LEVEL:	MILD	MODERATE	INTENSE
Workout schedule:	15–30 minutes, 3 times per week	30–45 minutes, 3–4 times per week	45–60 minutes, 4–5 times per week
Target heart rate:	15–25% maximum	25–50% maximum	50–65% maximum
Type of workout:	Walking, doing housework, climbing stairs, raking leaves, t'ai chi, yoga	Brisk walking or jogging, swimming, cycling, aerobics, team sports	Running, swimming, cycling, skiing, and other sports
Benefits:	• Increased energy levels	• Increased energy levels	• Increased energy levels

continued

ACTIVITY LEVEL:	MILD	MODERATE	INTENSE
	• Improved cardiovascular health and reduced risk of heart disease • Improved blood flow to the genitals • Weight loss	• Improved cardiovascular health and reduced risk of heart disease • Improved blood flow to genitals • Higher sex hormone levels resulting in boosted libido • Weight loss	• Improved cardiovascular health and reduced risk of heart disease • Improved blood flow to genitals • Boosted libido • Loss of body fat and increased muscle mass
Risks:	Very few	• Some chance of injury • Small risk of heart attack, especially in previously sedentary individuals	• Increased risk of injury and strain • Increased risk of heart attack among previously sedentary individuals

Weight

Now let's investigate the delicate relationship between weight and sexual fitness. This is no simple matter. Weight plays an important role in sexual functioning as well as body image and self-esteem. At the same time, when we discuss weight issues, realize that we are referring to a weight range that is considered by the medical establishment to be healthy for someone of your body type, age, and gender. We are not encouraging you to pursue Hollywood-type standards of "beauty" and thinness, but rather to consider the physiological consequences of being either severely over- or underweight. After all, the most important factor in terms of enjoying a satisfying sex life is being happy with who you are and how you look.

The media leads us to believe that in order to be sexual we must be young, beautiful, and thin. This is certainly not the case. In order to realize true sexual fitness, you must come to accept your body, to love it with all its unique characteristics. You need to view yourself as distinctive and special, not imperfect. You need to embrace yourself.

Just as fruits come in many different shapes—from the bottom-heavy form of a pear to the roundness of an apple to the long, thin banana—so do bodies. Body shape and size do not define our sexuality. A man with a few extra pounds of love handles is more attractive to women than one who obsesses over his weight. A woman who embraces her ample Rubenesque form is far sexier than someone who is model-thin but unhappy with who she is.

Another key factor to keep in mind is the difference between body fat and body size. Weight is a combination of the two. You cannot control your fundamental size. Whether you are big boned or small boned, tall or short has a basic impact on your weight, but you inherit this from your parents and ancestors. You can, however, control your body fat if you want to. While it depends partly on genetics, body fat can be affected by adapting your eating and exercise habits. Once you decide where you want to be in terms of body fat percentage, you can start working toward your goal.

> **FITNESS FACT**
>
> **Maintaining a weight beneficial to sexual fitness is a matter of balance—neither too much nor too little.**

It's important to figure out where your weight falls. There is a big difference between being a few pounds overweight and being clinically obese. The charts below will quickly help you to determine if you are within the recommended range, slightly overweight, severely overweight, or severely underweight. Real health issues arise when people fall into either of the two extreme categories. If you are in the appropriate to slightly overweight range and regularly see your doctor to ensure that you do not have high blood pressure, cholesterol, or other health problems, then you are probably fine.

Please note that these charts (which are prepared by the Metropolitan Life Insurance Company and are considered by some doctors to be too generous) provide you with only a fast, rough evaluation of your recommended weight range based on mortality rates. A far more accurate measure of your health risks takes into consideration your body fat percentage and activity level. For example, an athlete might

RECOMMENDED WEIGHT BASED ON HEIGHT—MEN

HEIGHT IN FEET & INCHES	SMALL FRAME	MEDIUM FRAME	LARGE FRAME
5'2"	128–134	131–141	138–150
5'3"	130–136	133–143	140–153
5'4"	132–138	135–145	142–156
5'5"	134–140	137–148	144–160
5'6"	136–142	139–151	146–164
5'7"	138–145	142–154	149–168
5'8"	140–148	145–157	152–172
5'9"	142–151	151–159	155–176
5'10"	144–154	153–163	158–180
5'11"	146–157	154–166	161–184
6'0"	149–160	157–170	164–188
6'1"	152–164	160–174	168–192
6'2"	155–168	165–178	172–197
6'3"	158–172	167–182	176–202
6'4"	162–176	171–187	181–207

RECOMMENDED WEIGHT BASED ON HEIGHT—WOMEN			
HEIGHT IN FEET & INCHES	SMALL FRAME	MEDIUM FRAME	LARGE FRAME
4'10"	102–111	109–121	118–131
4'11"	103–113	111–123	120–134
5'0"	104–115	113–126	122–137
5'1"	106–118	115–129	125–140
5'2"	108–121	118–132	128–143
5'3"	111–124	121–135	131–147
5'4"	114–127	124–138	134–151
5'5"	117–130	127–141	137–155
5'6"	120–133	130–144	140–159
5'7"	123–136	133–147	143–163
5'8"	126–139	136–150	146–167
5'9"	129–142	139–153	149–170
5'10"	132–145	142–156	152–173
5'11"	135–148	145–159	155–176
6'0"	138–151	148–162	158–179

technically have a weight-to-height ratio in the overweight range because of her dense, heavy muscle mass but not be at any risk for serious health problems. It is best to see your doctor or a nutritionist for a true determination of your ideal weight.

To use the tables above, first find your height on one of the two charts labeled "Recommended Weight Based on Height" depending on whether you are male or female. You should quickly be able to see if your weight is within the ideal range.

An alternative to the weight charts presented above is to calculate your body mass. The Body Mass Index (BMI) is a measurement highly

BMI RANGE			
WOMEN		MEN	
Less than 25	Ideal	Less than 26	Ideal
26–27	Borderline	27–28	Borderline
Greater than 27	Too high	Greater than 28	Too high

correlated with body fat, and is therefore considered a more accurate indication of obesity than body weight. Unfortunately, it's also a bit more difficult to calculate: Divide your weight in kilograms (kg) by your height in meters squared (m^2). For example, if you weigh 142 pounds (multiply by 0.45 = 64 kg) and are 5'9" tall (multiply height in inches by 0.025 = 1.75 m), your BMI is 21. Or just use the BMI calculator provided at www.sexualfitnessMD.com! The chart above indicates the ranges of BMI that are considered healthy and too high.

Being significantly underweight can pose serious health risks. It can lead to anemia, brittle bones, heart problems, fatigue, and other concerns. It can also jeopardize sexual function. A certain minimum level of body fat must be maintained in order to ensure normal hormone production. Low levels of key sex hormones mean that men and women who are severely underweight typically experience loss of libido and fertility.

Obesity can have both a physical and psychological impact on sexual fitness, as well. People who are severely overweight may have a negative body image, poor cardiovascular health, and unbalanced hormone levels. These factors all can detract from ability as well as desire to engage in sexual activity.

The good news is that if you are overweight, losing weight can significantly improve your sexual passion and performance. A clinical trial published in the *Journal of Obesity and Weight Regulation* revealed that when people lost enough weight to bring themselves to within ten pounds of their target weight, their level of sexual interest and activity rose substantially.

Making Exercise and Weight Work for You

For many people, being physically active on a regular basis and maintaining a healthy weight can pose a major challenge. However, you should feel encouraged by the scientific research presented here. It's important to remember that "regularly being active" does not mean that you must be an Olympic athlete. Nor does "maintaining a healthy weight" mean that you must be supermodel-thin. In fact, taking either weight or exercise to an extreme can prove destructive to your sexual vitality. What you should strive to achieve is moderation.

In terms of exercise, find a level and type of physical activity that is comfortable and enjoyable to you. That may mean a half-hour walk in the woods every day, a game of golf a few times a week, or some combination of the two. Keep yourself interested and excited by variability.

In terms of weight, it's best not to obsess. Read the weight charts provided here, but talk with your doctor to determine the appropriate weight range for you given a variety of factors including your age, activity level, genetic background, and gender. Also, there are many resources for you to draw on, from community centers, to weight management programs, to on-line support groups. Feel free to seek out assistance.

Whatever you do, try not to agonize over every calorie you eat or every pound you lose. Aim at making lifestyle changes rather than following crash diets. It's worth your while: weight lost suddenly is frequently regained. And remember that all the components of the Sexual Fitness Program, including being more active, eating a well-balanced diet, and caring for your body, will serve to help you manage your weight as well as to enhance your sexual vitality.

Most important, listen to your body. Society has many unrealistic expectations of how thin and how athletic we should be. The point of sexual fitness is for you to reach your full potential in terms of sexual drive, pleasure, and performance, as well as general health. Therefore, the best solution is to set personal goals for yourself based on what *you* want to achieve, then go for it!

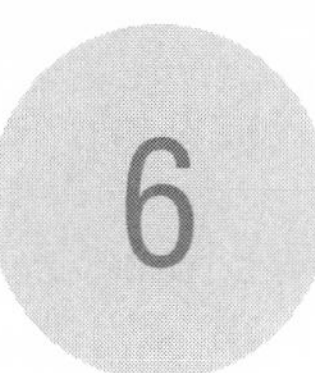

Sleep

> Blessings on him who invented sleep—the mantle that covers all human thoughts, the food that appeases hunger, the drink that quenches thirst, the fire that warms cold, the cold that moderates heat.
>
> —MIGUEL DE CERVANTES

Most of us at some point have felt the deadening effects of fatigue on our sex lives. With our busy schedules, it is typical for people to feel too tired for sex. Sleep deprivation is devastating to sexual fitness. When you lack sleep, your interest in many activities—including sex—severely declines. So do your testosterone levels. In addition, abnormal sleeping patterns are associated with an increased risk of infertility. When you get plenty of sleep, on the other hand, you are more likely to stay healthy and maintain a positive outlook on life. Adequate rest helps your body recover from illness and injury. And yet even though doctors recommend getting eight hours of sleep a night, 43 percent of Americans say they usually sleep only six or fewer hours.

It is important to sleep according to a regular nightly schedule because, otherwise, we upset our circadian rhythms. Circadian rhythms are the natural cycle of sleep and wakefulness that serve as the body's biological clock. They follow a predictable pattern, regulating your body temperature, metabolism, and hormone levels throughout a twenty-four-hour period. They can affect your appetite, athletic performance, and sexual function. Your rhythms are naturally set according to the sun, regardless of the hours you keep. For example, testosterone levels peak in the morning for men. So when you get out of sync with your biological clock—through irregular sleep patterns, working nights, or traveling across time zones—your ability to sleep well, your sexual fitness, and your general health all may suffer.

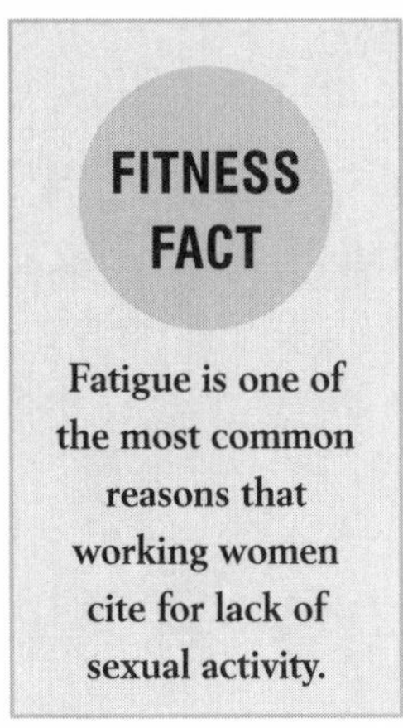

In this chapter, you'll see how sleeping better can make you feel and perform better—at work, at home, and in bed. And the good news is that "sleeping better" does not necessarily mean you need to increase the number of hours you sleep each night. You may benefit simply from improving the quality of your sleep. We suggest keeping a sleep calendar that will assist you in determining whether or not you're getting enough sleep. Then we discuss some of the most common factors that interfere with healthy sleep patterns. You'll also find suggestions for making sure that you enjoy deep, sound sleep as often as possible.

How Much Is Enough?

Most people need about eight hours of sleep a night. That is just an average, not a hard-and-fast rule. The truth is that everyone's body is a little different. You probably know people who must sleep nine hours a night or they turn into cranky monsters and others who never seem to need more than six hours to keep their engines firing. (Nevertheless, if you're regularly getting less than five hours a night you should see a physician because you may have a serious physical or psychological condition that is interfering with your ability to sleep). Sleep requirements vary by person, but how do you determine the optimal amount of sleep for *you*?

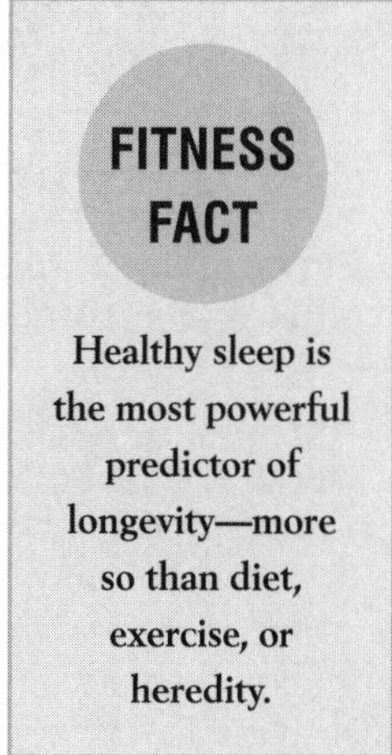

Healthy sleep is the most powerful predictor of longevity—more so than diet, exercise, or heredity.

You can start by figuring out whether or not you're sleep deprived and adding on hours from there. One quick way to test sleep deprivation is to track the amount of time between when you climb into bed and when you fall asleep. Despite what you may have heard, you shouldn't nod off the second your head hits the pillow. Rather, if you're well rested, you ought to lie awake for about fifteen minutes before drifting into slumber. Losing consciousness immediately is a sure sign that you're not getting enough sleep. Other signs of sleep deprivation may include a tendency to fall asleep during the day when you're at meetings and other low-activity-level events, an unusual irritability toward others, and significantly greater than normal difficulty concentrating or remembering facts.

You can also determine if you're sleep deprived by testing yourself on the Stanford Sleepiness Scale (SSS), shown on the next page. Your level of alertness will naturally vary throughout the day according to your circadian rhythm. Generally, people feel most awake around 9 A.M. and 9 P.M., with their alertness level dipping at about 3 o'clock in the afternoon. However, you should never feel drowsy all day, nor should you ever feel as if you must go to sleep at once. Measure your sleepiness, according to the scale, at various points throughout the day while you're engaged in different activities: when you wake up first thing in the morning, at about 10 A.M., at lunch, during an afternoon meeting or work session, and in the evening around dinnertime. If you consistently score below a 3 on the SSS, then you're probably not getting enough sound sleep.

THE STANFORD SLEEPINESS SCALE	
DEGREE OF SLEEPINESS	**SCALE RATING**
Feeling active, vital, alert, or wide-awake	1
Functioning at high levels, but not at peak; able to concentrate	2
Awake but relaxed; responsive but not fully alert	3
Somewhat foggy, let down	4
Foggy; losing interest in remaining awake; slowed down	5
Sleepy, woozy, fighting sleep; prefer to lie down	6
No longer fighting sleep, sleep onset soon; having dreamlike thoughts	7
Asleep	X

Another way to ensure that you're getting enough sleep is to determine your personal sleep requirement. As we discussed earlier, each person has his or her own optimum amount of sleep per night. On the following page, you'll find a work sheet for tracking your sleep patterns. Choose a calm week when you are either on vacation or don't have anything particularly stressful going on in your life for completing this exercise. Try to go to bed at the same time every night, but allow yourself to fall asleep and wake up whenever you like. All week, you need to avoid setting an alarm, taking any sleep aids, or worrying about oversleeping. It's also important that you not consume alcohol, cigarettes, caffeine, or any stimulants after 4 P.M. Now all you need do is to record how many hours you sleep and when. At the end of the week, examine your sleep pattern. What is your body's natural inclination? Nine hours? Six? Whatever it is, strive for approximately that amount of sleep every day because it's what your body needs.

Also, notice at what time you naturally tend to fall asleep and wake up. Some people are night owls who thrive on staying up late, whereas others can't stay awake past early evening and then wake with the sun. Whatever your body's preference, try to stick to that sleeping pattern if your schedule permits. You'll be amazed at how much more energetic you feel when you work with your body instead of against it.

SLEEP CALENDAR

	MON.	TUES.	WED.	THURS.	FRI.	SAT.	SUN.
Time to bed							
Time asleep							
Time awake (w/o alarm)							
Total hours of sleep							
Energy level upon waking (Refreshed/Somewhat refreshed/fatigued)							
Energy level throughout day (Refreshed/Somewhat refreshed/fatigued)							

Just as important as the amount of sleep you get is the quality of that sleep. Not all sleep is of equal value. In order to reap the full benefits of your precious resting hours, you need to sleep soundly and keep nighttime awakenings to a minimum. Only by reaching the deepest levels of sleep will you ensure yourself a totally refreshed feeling upon waking.

The Effects of Sleep Deprivation

Sleep deprivation has a direct impact on your sexual activity. It can cause a decline in sex drive, testosterone levels, and fertility. It is also associated with a depressed mood and negative state of mind, which serve to detract from sexual interest, pleasure, and performance.

Take Susan, for example. Susan is always tired. She gets up at the crack of dawn to go for a brisk walk, her only chance to exercise during her busy days. By the time she returns, her two children, aged six and ten, are already climbing out of bed. With the assistance of her husband, Tom, she helps the kids get ready, feeds them, and sends them off to school. Two hours after waking, she finally begins her "real work"—her job. She spends the day managing her boss, dealing with last-minute demands, and balancing ten tasks at once in her hectic career as a personal assistant.

When Susan finishes work, she already feels ready for bed. But she still has to pick up her children from the baby-sitter and help them with their homework, figure out what to do about dinner, and take care of some personal errands. If she's lucky, she has a few minutes to spend with Tom after bathing the kids and putting them to bed. She likes to just lie in bed and talk before drifting off to sleep. Susan wonders how, at the end of a typical day, she could possibly have enough energy for sex.

Your body's natural instinct is to shut off sex when you are fatigued. After all, why would Nature want you to reproduce when you're not taking care of yourself? In several clinical trials, healthy men who were deprived of sleep for forty-eight-hour periods experienced a significant drop in testosterone levels. Once they resumed normal sleeping patterns, testosterone levels rose. As we've discussed in previous chapters, low testosterone levels are strongly correlated with low levels of sexual desire and activity. One study revealed that 44 percent of people with sleep-disordered breathing (e.g., sleep apnea, chronic snoring), a condition that prevents them from getting a restful night's sleep, suffer from decreased libido and/or erectile dysfunction (ED).

Fertility is also affected by sleeping patterns. Sleeping irregular hours can lower a woman's chances of having a successful pregnancy. A study of infertility conducted in seven European countries revealed that women who worked night shifts took significantly longer to become pregnant than did women in the general population. Many other studies have discovered a correlation between night-shift work and unfavorable pregnancy outcomes, including spontaneous abortion, pregnancy loss, premature birth, and low birth weight. Researchers believe that working nights or sleeping irregular hours has a negative impact on fertility because it disrupts normal daily hormonal patterns, which operate according to circadian rhythms.

In addition, sleep deprivation alters your psychological state of mind, a crucial factor in terms of sexual fitness. A study of college students found a strong correlation between high-quality sleep and overall health and sense of well-being. People with insomnia, on the other hand, are more likely to suffer from anxiety and depression. Psychological issues of this nature detract from a healthy sex life: when you're not feeling good about yourself and the world, you're less likely to be interested in sexual intimacy.

Insomnia

Forty-eight percent of Americans say that they experience insomnia occasionally, and almost one-quarter claim to suffer from it every night. Insomnia refers to difficulty falling asleep or staying asleep, poor sleep quality, or waking up not feeling refreshed. It can last from a few days to a few weeks or even longer. It can be caused by a variety of factors including health problems, menopause, psychological stress, and lifestyle issues such as frequent travel. The good news is that, in most cases, there are solutions for combating insomnia and improving your sleep life.

Physical Health Issues

Insomnia may result from sleep-disordered breathing, a category of sleep-related health conditions that includes chronic snoring. In terms of sexual fitness and general health, obstructive sleep apnea (OSA) is the most serious and disruptive type of sleep-disordered breathing. OSA is characterized by snoring, periods of halted breathing, frequent awakenings, and excessive daytime sleepiness. People suffering from OSA may experience memory loss, disordered thinking, anxiety, and depression. In fact, many patients suffering from OSA report low libido or sexual dysfunction. These sexual side effects probably result from the chronic fatigue, depression, and unbalanced hormone levels caused by OSA.

Other types of physical problems can interfere with sleep, as well. Pain from chronic illnesses, such as arthritis or cancer, can make restful sleep very difficult to achieve. Unfortunately, medications don't always help. Prescription and over-the-counter drugs for depression, asthma, high blood pressure, and even the common cold (antihistamines) can keep you awake by stimulating your energy levels or making you feel nervous.

If you have any trouble sleeping due to physical factors, including sleep-disordered breathing, you should see a doctor. Many of these problems can be treated. Also, be sure to ask if any medicines that you take on a regular basis have sleep-altering side effects.

Menopause

Insomnia is a common problem for many postmenopausal women. As women age, their estrogen levels naturally tend to decline. Low estrogen levels can lead to hot flashes, which frequently disturb women's ability to sleep soundly, causing them to wake during the night in an agitated and overheated state.

Fortunately, there is a potential solution for many women. Estrogen replacement therapy (ERT) has proven effective in helping women at menopause to overcome their sleep problems. ERT reduces hot flashes, enhances the quality of sleep, and decreases the frequency of nighttime arousal. However, ERT does have certain risks, so be sure to carefully consider this option with your doctor. (For more information on ERT, see chapter 3: *Medications*.)

Psychological Stress

Stress steals sleep. In fact, insomnia is a very common side effect of anxiety and depression. In one European survey, both men and women claimed that, more than anything else, the stress and worries of everyday life, such as work pressure, interpersonal problems, and family discord, caused them to lose sleep.

If you're looking for ways to reduce stress, read on. In chapter 7: *Stress Reduction*, you'll find information and specific activities designed to help you take control of the stress in your life. You'll also find many suggestions of simple things you can do to help yourself sleep better in the next section, "Improving Your Sleep Habits." For example, you might take a hot bath before bed or trade massages with your partner.

Lifestyle Factors

Without even realizing it, you may be doing things every day that harm your ability to get a sound night's sleep. Some common culprits include smoking; drinking alcohol in the evening; sleeping in an uncomfortable, disruptive environment; and napping too much. (See the next section for helpful hints on improving your daily sleep habits.) You might also travel frequently.

Traveling across more than two time zones will interfere with your natural sleep cycle. It confuses your body's internal clock, upsetting circadian rhythms. As a result, many frequent business travelers suffer from jet lag, a phenomenon characterized by falling asleep in the middle of the afternoon and waking up in the wee hours of the morning. If you travel often, you should be aware that you might be suffering the effects of sleep deprivation.

Your body typically needs several days to recover from jet lag. Here are some suggestions for how you can speed the adaptation process:

- Adjust your sleep pattern forward or back by several hours a few days before departing on your trip in anticipation of the new time zone.
- Set your watch to the new time as soon as you get on the plane. The sooner you accept the new time zone as the one you're living in, the better.
- Take a flight that arrives in the early evening, then force yourself to stay awake until at least 10 P.M. Try to avoid flights that arrive early in the morning, as you'll have difficulty staying awake throughout the day.
- Allow yourself to nap for only brief periods while adjusting to the new time zone. Long naps will tell your body that it's nighttime, when in reality it's daytime.
- Get outdoors as frequently as possible when you arrive, as sunlight will help reset your biological clock.

Sleeping Pills

Sleeping medications can prove beneficial to certain people in certain situations. They are generally recommended if insomnia occurs because of a specific physical problem (e.g., PMS) or event (e.g., an upcoming speech) and is known to be short-term, or if the person has not responded to behavioral therapy. Hypnotics, or sedatives, as they are known in scientific terms, can diminish the amount of time it takes a person to fall asleep, result in longer periods of more sound sleep, reduce the number of nighttime awakenings, and generally help you feel less distressed.

However, taking sleeping pills can be detrimental to your sexual fitness and general health. Benzodiazepine sedatives, the most commonly prescribed type of sleeping pills, can interfere with sexual desire and response. These changes occur as a result of the sedation, muscle relaxation, depressed mood, and lack of attention that frequently accompany hypnotics use. For example, muscle relaxation may make it more difficult to reach orgasm. Another type of sedative, zolpidem (brand name Ambien), which is not a benzodiazepine, may have fewer sexual side effects, but evidence is not clear at this time.

Most doctors believe that sleeping pills should not be taken over the long term as many people develop tolerance to them over time and some people may even become addicted. Sleeping pills can also cause unpleasant side effects such as daytime sleepiness, inattention, and forgetfulness. In addition, they may interfere with breathing, making problems worse for people already suffering from insomnia due to sleep apnea. Sleeping pills should be used only occasionally or nightly for a very short period of time. They should never be taken in combination with alcohol or other sedatives.

Improving Your Sleep Habits

Optimum general and sexual health requires adequate sleep quantity and quality. It doesn't matter if you get nine hours of sleep at night but are awakened every hour—you won't feel rested in the morning. For a satisfying and beneficial rest, you need to reduce the number of times you wake up during the night. Being "awake" may mean reaching semiconsciousness for just a few seconds. You may not even be aware that something is disturbing you, yet you are pulled out of the deepest sleep stages that are so necessary for feeling refreshed the next day. So how do you cut back on rude awakenings?

Here are tips from the experts on how to get to sleep and stay asleep—without the help of medications. For peak energy and libido, make these habits part of your sexual fitness routine.

1. Stick to a steady sleep schedule.

Go to bed and get up at the same time every day. Continue to get up on schedule even on weekends. You'll be surprised to find that, after a week or so, you won't even need an alarm clock. Your body will be delighted to know what to expect, and you'll reap the rewards by sleeping more soundly every night.

2. Beware of napping.

If you have any trouble sleeping at night, you should avoid napping during the day. Although it may make you feel good in the short term, in the long term napping will interfere with your ability to establish a routine sleep schedule. However, if you are a sound sleeper who only needs a nap occasionally to boost energy, then go for it. Just make sure to limit yourself to no more than thirty minutes of napping a day.

3. Establish a bedtime ritual.

Instead of just jumping into bed at the end of a busy day, prepare yourself for sleep with a calming ritual. Many people enjoy reading or listening to music. You might also try taking a shower or bath: hot water eases the transition into deep sleep by changing your body temperature. Other options include cuddling with your partner or meditating. The specific activity you choose does not matter as much as the fact that doing it helps you to relax and clear your mind. A lot of people say that having sex is the perfect way to ensure a pleasant, restful night's sleep!

4. Keep your bedroom sacred.

Make sure that you use your bedroom *only* for sleeping and having sex. Do not use it to do work, fight, worry, watch TV, or even talk on the phone. When you do, you create associations for yourself between the bedroom and stress, making it more difficult for you to get in the mood for sex or to fall asleep there. By reserving your bedroom for only activities conducive to sleep and sex, you will keep it a positive space that always makes you feel good. You'll associate it only with pleasurable activities.

Even if you have a one-room apartment or work from home, you can seal off the area immediately around your bed with a curtain or screen. If you have more space, move all work-related items such as computer and desk, and even television and VCR, out of the room completely. If you start stressing out while lying in bed at night, get up and move to a different room until you are sleepy.

5. Ensure that your pillow and mattress are comfortable.

Common sense says that if you're constantly tossing and turning in an attempt to get comfy, you'll never get a sound night's sleep. There is no magic formula for how hard or soft your bedding should be—all that matters is that it feels good to you. When purchasing new pillows and mattresses, take your time checking them out in the store. Lie on them for a good five minutes straight—even if you feel as if you're making a fool of yourself.

Look for neck-support pillows—pillows that conform to the contours of your head and neck. These pillows are formed to support your head and neck at an angle parallel to the bed, with no forward or backward tilt. In a clinical study, when people slept with neck-support pillows they reported more sound quality sleep than when sleeping with regular pillows. You can purchase these pillows at most bedding stores.

Your mattress should evenly distribute your body weight. You want to avoid placing undue pressure on your shoulders, hips, or other body parts. A good mattress salesperson should be able to help you find the one that best suits your sleeping position and body type. Also, if you share a bed with a partner, remember that bigger is better. The larger the mattress, the less likely you are to feel your bedmate's nighttime tossing and turning.

If you are not sleeping well on your current bed, check for lumps and sags. Don't sleep on a mattress that's deteriorated into something unrecognizable—buy a new one. Another option is to purchase a foam pad or feather bed that adds some extra cushioning. Don't shy away from making a real investment in your pillow and mattress. Even though we spend one-third of our lives sleeping, we rarely change our bedding!

6. Minimize noise.

All through the night dogs bark and car alarms sound. It's pretty apparent that loud, sudden noises can wake you up. But did you know that sounds can disturb your sleep even if you're not aware of them? Remember that you only need to rise to a state of semiconsciousness in order to upset your sleep cycles.

Block out environmental noise. It's possible to reduce the sound conductivity of your room by furnishing it with double-paned glass, carpets, and heavy drapes. You might also consider wearing earplugs, playing soft, relaxing music in the background, or purchasing a noisemaker if necessary. These inexpensive machines can generate the sounds of surf, rainfall, crickets, a heartbeat, or simply white noise. Air conditioners and purification systems can sometimes also produce a pleasant background hum that you can use to cover up the sounds of the outside world.

7. Control your exposure to light.

Sunlight is the most powerful regulator of the sleep/wake cycle. Your body is trained through millions of years of evolution to respond to the sun. You detect daylight even through closed eyelids. So if you get up later than the sun does, you need to keep light out of your bedroom. Either fit your room with heavy curtains or wear a sleep mask. Otherwise you'll be waking with the sun at 6 A.M., even subconsciously.

If you work nights or live in a climate where the sun rarely appears, you may want to consider exposing yourself to artificial light during the day. Not spending enough time in the sun could be interfering with your ability to sleep. Sun visors are available at specialty sleep stores and on the Internet. (Please note: they are not the same as sun-tanning beds.) These visors provide light, tricking your body into thinking that it is sunny outside. In a clinical trial, women over the age of sixty-five wore sun visors for thirty minutes every day for two weeks. During and even after the study period, the women demonstrated a significant increase in sleep duration and quality. Be aware, however, that sun visors should only be used with a doctor's supervision.

Once you are ready to get up, sleep researchers recommend spending at least twenty minutes in the sun. Doing so will help set your body clock to the new day and keep you on a regular sleeping schedule. Also, sunlight suppresses production of melatonin, the hormone that makes us want to fall asleep at night.

8. Maintain satisfactory room temperature.

Obviously you won't sleep well if you are either too hot or too cold. Make sure that your room stays at a comfortable temperature throughout the night. Experts say that the optimal temperature for sleeping is a cool 65 degrees. When your bedroom is too warm, your sleep is disrupted. Hot rooms increase nighttime awakenings and prevent you from drifting happily into the deepest levels of sleep.

9. Exercise early in the day.

Regular exercise is one of the best ways to ensure sound sleep. It tires out your muscles and fatigues your body in a healthy way, allowing you to relax more easily. Most people who exercise feel that it has a greater positive impact on sleep than any single other factor, including a good day at work or a quiet sleeping environment. In a clinical trial of people aged fifty to seventy-six published in the *Journal of the American Medical Association,* those who followed an exercise regimen slept better and longer than did a control group. Exercise has also been proven an effective treatment for sleep disorders. And let's not forget the benefits of exercise to sexual fitness!

However, you need to plan when you work out to best enhance your sleep. If you exercise late in the evening, you may not be tired enough by bedtime to fall asleep. When you work out, your body temperature rises and you secrete adrenaline, a stimulant. In other words, you literally "pump yourself up." Exercising at night (three to four hours before bedtime) can delay sleep by up to forty minutes. So, to reap the maximum benefit of your workout routine, try to work out at least six hours before you go to bed.

10. Stay away from stimulants.

If you want to sleep, why pump yourself full of chemicals that make you stay awake? It's best not to consume stimulants within six hours of when you plan to go to bed. Caffeine not only makes you feel more alert but also increases your need to urinate, meaning more frequent nighttime trips to the bathroom. So avoid that afternoon latte with a friend—or make it a decaf. Remember that many types of tea, cola, and even hot chocolate contain caffeine, as well.

Nicotine is another stimulant. As a result of their nicotine intake, smokers tend to have problems going to sleep and staying asleep, and report high levels of daytime sleepiness. In addition, cigarette smoking is associated with snoring, probably because it interferes with breathing. People who quit smoking, on the other hand, report that they fall asleep more easily and wake less often during the night. Of course, smoking has a direct negative impact on sexual fitness, as well. This offers yet another great incentive to kick the habit.

11. Refrain from using alcohol to fall asleep.

Do you ever have a glass of alcohol to help yourself doze off when you can't fall asleep? If you drink, you're probably familiar with the way that alcohol induces drowsiness. Alcohol is, in fact, a sedative. As a result, many people like to have a nightcap to relax, thinking it will help them sleep better. But this is not the case at all. In fact, alcohol causes abnormal sleep patterns. It interferes with the deepest periods of sleep that are crucial to feeling refreshed in the morning. What's more, alcohol has what's called a "rebound effect," which means that it often causes people to awaken in the early-morning hours. So skip the drinks after 7 P.M. if you want to ensure a sound night's sleep. And remember that having more than one to two glasses of alcohol will interfere with sexual performance, as well.

12. Moderate your late-night consumption of food and beverages.

Try to avoid eating large, heavy meals close to bedtime. If you feel "stuffed" when you go to bed, you'll likely have trouble falling asleep. What's more, lying down aggravates heartburn. You may end up tossing and turning in discomfort throughout the night. On the other hand, hunger pangs can keep you awake. Rather than going to bed starving, enjoy a small snack as you retire for the evening. Your best option is a food high in protein and low in carbohydrates, such as a handful of nuts, as it will satisfy your hunger but not make you feel overly full.

Also, restrict your consumption of beverages just before bedtime. With too much fluid in your stomach, you'll end up awakening frequently to use the bathroom.

13. Warm your feet.

Body temperature plays a critical role in regulating sleep. Scientists theorize that the simple act of lying down may induce sleepiness by redistributing blood—and therefore body heat—from the core to the peripheral areas of your body. They've recently discovered that you can regulate your body temperature and control your sleepiness by keeping your feet warm at night. In one study, warm feet proved more effective in putting a group of men to sleep than did treatment with light or melatonin. Researchers suggest keeping your feet warm with an old-fashioned hot-water bottle or socks. They especially recommend this practice for the elderly, who tend to have poor circulation and, therefore, cold feet.

14. Get a massage.

Studies conducted at the University of Miami School of Medicine's Touch Research Institute reveal that massage helps people sleep better. It works by turning off the sympathetic nervous system, responsible for stimulating our "fight or flight" response, and turning on the parasympathetic nervous system, responsible for calming us down. A massaged body is more relaxed, less tense, and better able to slip off into slumber.

15. Consider trying supplements.

As we discussed earlier, although sleeping pills are helpful for certain people in certain situations, they can also prove detrimental to your general and sexual health. If you're suffering from a bout of insomnia, having a particularly stressful week, or experiencing jet lag, you might consider trying a natural sleep aid. Valerian and melatonin are two popular options, which many people claim are effective.

The root of the valerian plant has been used in Ayurvedic and traditional Chinese medicine for thousands of years. Valerian purportedly improves sleep without the mind-numbing side effects of sleeping pills. People who take valerian claim that it improves both the quality of their sleep and ease in falling asleep. Take the dose recommended by the manufacturer about an hour before bedtime.

Melatonin is another sleep aid. This naturally occurring hormone regulates sleepiness, with levels in our bodies about six times higher at night than during the day. We produce it in response to darkness. Levels of the hormone decline with age. Many people use melatonin to fight jet lag, as well as to alleviate sleep disorders due to aging, shift work, and chronic insomnia. If you're interested, try taking 2 to 3 mg about thirty minutes before bedtime.

Sleeping Together

Couples may have particular issues with sleeping soundly through the night if they share a bed. Here are a few suggestions for improving your joint sleeping arrangement.

A. Sleep in a large bed with an extra-firm mattress.

One of the most annoying factors in sharing a bed is being awakened by your partner's tossing and turning. In order to avoid being disturbed by these nighttime movements, sleep on a large, extra-firm mattress. There are even mattresses specially designed to keep your body movements totally isolated to your section of the bed.

B. Arrange for individual temperature control.

Another common problem is temperature: one person likes to sleep cold, another likes to sleep hot. There are ways to compromise so that you both enjoy a sound night's sleep. Generally, you'll need to keep the room cool enough to satisfy both of you. The person who needs the extra warmth can then sleep with additional blankets or wear heavier pajamas and socks. You can even purchase an electric blanket with separate temperature controls for each side of the bed.

C. Don't sleep in the same bed.

Some couples find that their sleeping habits are incompatible. Here's a way for you to sleep on separate beds while still sharing the intimacy of sleeping "together." Simply push two twin beds next to each other! That way, you'll each have your own mattress and blankets. You'll each be in total control of sleep temperature and you won't feel each other's fitful movements, but you will still be able to grab your lover's hand or cuddle just before you fall asleep.

Now that you have these secrets for sound slumber, put them to good use. Sleep is a healthy habit that is easy to neglect. When we get busy, we often tell ourselves, "Well, I can always stay up late to get this done." But the next time you're struggling with sleep deprivation, remind yourself why sleep is so crucial to your sexual fitness.

When you get an adequate amount of sleep every night, you feel good about yourself and have more energy. Your outlook on life improves. You feel rested. You can handle problems more easily. Your sex drive, sexual performance, and fertility are in better condition. Even with all the demands you have on your time, you have to admit that those are pretty convincing reasons to make sure you're getting enough sleep on a regular basis. Treat your body as it deserves to be treated. It is like a precious treasure, and the only one you'll ever have.

7 Stress Reduction

Everyone is stressed-out these days. Literally. According to an *American Demographics* poll, six in ten adults in the United States say they feel under great stress at least once a week. The hectic pace of modern life, with ever-increasing responsibilities, new technology, and little time for ourselves, places a burden on all of us.

Chronic stress can be devastating to your overall wellness and can also interfere with your sex life. When people are stressed, sexual intimacy is often the first thing to go because it involves the time and energy, cooperation and interest of two individuals. According to a survey in the *Journal of the American Medical Association*, stress is highly correlated with problems such as erectile dysfunction (ED) and performance anxiety in men, arousal difficulties and anorgasmia (the inability to reach orgasm) in women, and lack of libido in both sexes.

A scientist and stress expert, Dr. Robert Sapolsky, says that humans simply did not evolve to be able to cope with the constant daily stress of our modern lives. When our ancestors were hunter-gatherers, their main concerns were finding food and avoiding man-eating tigers or hostile neighborhood tribes—in other words, survival. In case of attack, the "fight or flight" response played a powerful, life-saving role. When it kicked in, it would immediately boost people's bodies into high gear, enabling them to perform extraordinary physical and mental tasks. During these sporadic periods of stress, the body would automatically shut off tasks like eating and digestion, sex and reproduction—anything that was secondary to making it through that moment alive.

The problem is that in today's world we tend to have the fight-or-flight reaction all the time, and to stimuli that act nothing like a man-eating tiger. We stress out about gaining weight, running out of cash, not performing well at work, the computer crashing, sitting in traffic, speaking in front of a large group of people, and running late. Although we do not need to be nearly as concerned about day-to-day survival as were our ancestors, we do have more time to dwell on success, career, money, and other anxiety-creating issues. Plus, whereas shopping at the supermarket is easier than killing live animals (or maybe it isn't!), we also deal with a far more complex world than the hunter-gatherers ever did.

So instead of being an occasional, life-saving reaction to extreme physical danger, stress today is often a nearly constant, undesirable reaction to psychological conflict. We get stressed-out when life feels out of control or when we perceive a threat to our well-being, confidence, efficiency, or happiness. As a result, the stress response kicks in far more frequently than nature ever intended. That's why, according to Dr. Sapolsky, zebras don't get ulcers but people do.

The good news is that you can manage stress; you don't have to let it manage you. You can teach yourself to view stress in a different light. If you believe you are in charge, then you will be. You can't control everything that happens to you, but you can determine your reactions. The one thing you can truly control in life is your attitude.

You can also adopt a lifestyle that is conducive to optimum sexual and general health, which includes getting plenty of rest, making time for yourself, exercising, and eating a healthy diet (all elements of the Sexual Fitness Program). Doing so will ensure that you are in the best possible physical and mental condition to deal with stress. Finally, you can benefit from practicing stress-reduction techniques like the ones recommended later in this chapter, such as meditation, massage, and aromatherapy. Taking simple steps such as these will help you achieve balance and reduce the impact of stress on your daily life.

How Stressed Are You?

Given the potential harm that stress can do to your sexual fitness, you're probably wondering if you're overstressed. We all suffer a certain degree of stress in our lives, but when is it too much? Here is a list of typical symptoms of chronic stress to watch out for:

- You find that stress is regularly interfering with your ability to get things done.
- You feel overwhelmed.
- You are irritable and snap at people more often than normal.
- You experience mood swings for no particular reason.
- You are tired most or all of the time and don't have the energy you usually have.
- You cry easily.
- You have difficulty concentrating on the task at hand.
- You lack motivation.
- You have trouble sleeping: you can't fall asleep, have trouble staying asleep, or wake up very early.
- You don't have your usual appetite.
- You feel depressed, anxious, or worried all the time.
- You develop physical problems such as upset stomach, diarrhea, heart palpitations, or excessive sweating and shaking.

If you believe that you are suffering from chronic stress, don't despair. You can develop healthy lifestyle habits and practice specific techniques designed to help you take control of your life.

The Effects of Stress

Both acute (temporary, immediate responses to events) and chronic (the long-term, cumulative load of minor day-to-day issues) stress can interfere with your sex life. Most people recognize the fact that stress makes them less interested in sex. Have you ever noticed how much better the sex is when you are on vacation? And how little you want to invest energy in sexual activity after a long, exhausting day at work? We all know that stress can make us feel drained and distracted. What you may not know, however, is that stress impairs sexual fitness on both the psychological and physiological levels.

Physiological Consequences

Stress directly affects sexual fitness in several ways. It can potentially interfere with male erections and female sexual arousal, cause a drop in libido, and reduce fertility.

Acute stress restricts blood flow to the genitals, which hinders physiological arousal. A stressful event—whether in the form of a car accident, a missed meeting, conflict in the workplace, or unhappy news—invokes the fight-or-flight response. When this happens, your nervous system is activated and your adrenal glands release the stress hormone adrenaline into your body. Adrenaline causes your heart rate to rise and your blood vessels to constrict so that blood is delivered to where it's needed—the muscles, and not the genitals. This response can save your life in case of crisis by enabling you to move more quickly and powerfully, but it inhibits male erections and female sexual arousal. During and immediately after a jolting, stressful event, adrenaline actually prevents men from being able to achieve or sustain erections.

Over time, chronic stress may also interfere with male erections and female sexual arousal by causing cholesterol levels to rise, exacerbating arteriosclerosis, or hardening of the arteries. As we've discussed in previous chapters, anything that harms the cardiovascular system is bad news for sexual fitness, because narrowed arteries mean restricted blood flow through the tiny arteries of the genitals.

Furthermore, stress causes a drop in testosterone levels and, therefore, libido. A threatening or anxiety-producing event causes the adrenal glands to secrete the stress hormone cortisol. Cortisol stimulates the body's metabolism but also suppresses production of testosterone. As we've discussed before, low testosterone levels are correlated with reduced sexual interest, drive, fantasy, and behavior. Lack of testosterone due to chronic stress may also result in impaired fertility in men. In a study of men at a fertility clinic, sperm concentration and total number of active sperm decreased significantly when self-reported stress increased.

Chronic stress appears to suppress fertility in women, as well. In the first place, it may upset the menstrual cycle. It is quite common for women to stop menstruating when going through a stressful life period, such as beginning college or starting a new job. Women who work in jobs they consider to be stressful tend to have less-regular menstrual cycles than do women who work in jobs that they consider low-anxiety. Scientists speculate that this phenomenon occurs because stress causes production of key hormones involved in reproduction to decline.

In addition, stress appears to increase the risk of unfavorable pregnancy outcomes. A study of Thai women found that working long hours (more than seventy-one hours per week) increased the time it took them to conceive. An article published in *Fertility and Sterility* revealed that women who rated themselves as under a great deal of stress were twelve times more likely to miscarry early in their pregnancies than were less-stressed women.

Psychological Consequences

It's a stressful time in your life. You are worried about finances or have been frustrated with work. Although in general you feel satisfied with your relationship with your partner, you notice that your sex life has really suffered. You feel anxious and depressed, and so rarely find yourself in the mood for intimacy. Once you are engaged in sexual activity, you can't concentrate on being with your lover because your mind keeps drifting. Your partner becomes frustrated with you, and this only makes you feel more stressed-out.

Stress does more than interfere with your physical ability to perform. It also affects your state of mind. Chronic stress often leads to depression, anxiety, and distracting thoughts, all of which detract from sexual passion, pleasure, and performance.

How does stress contribute to depression? It lowers brain levels of serotonin and dopamine, neurotransmitters responsible for keeping you in a good mood. Dopamine is critical to sex drive, so low levels of the neurotransmitter often mean a decline in sexual interest along with depression. These physiological factors can stimulate a vicious cycle whereby excess stress leads to depression, which leads to lack of sexual desire, which then adds to the level of stress in a person's life and further contributes to depression.

Stress also creates anxiety. Chronic anxiety—the kind that results from daily worries—permanently raises stress hormone levels, which can interfere with performance, make it more difficult to become aroused, and lower libido.

Finally, stress tends to fill the mind with distracting, worrying thoughts. Scientific research has revealed that when people are distracted they don't become as sexually aroused. In several clinical trials, the more subjects needed to concentrate on complicated tasks, the less they responded to erotic stimuli. Both erections in men and sexual arousal in women suffered. In addition, participants reported that, subjectively, they felt less interested in sex when distracted.

Stress Reduction

In order to enjoy sexual fitness to the fullest, it is important to be able to relieve stress and even find ways to escape it completely from time to time. Remember that stress can cause a decrease in sexual drive, arousal, and performance by affecting you on both the physiological and psychological levels. When you actively manage stress, on the other hand, you optimize your sexual potential.

In this section, you will find numerous suggestions for stress reduction, so do what works best for you. Engaging in even a simple exercise such as buying flowers for your room and noting their beauty can help you make a difference. Decide now that you are going to manage stress instead of letting it control you, and you'll enjoy the effects for the rest of your life. You will not always feel calm and relaxed—no one can achieve that state. On the road of life, we all need to confront major obstacles and crises that make us feel overwhelmed and anxious, and may even have an impact on our sexuality. But it is your ability to handle stress that will determine how positive you feel, how healthy you remain, and how sexually fit you become. Stress management can change the way you live from this day forward.

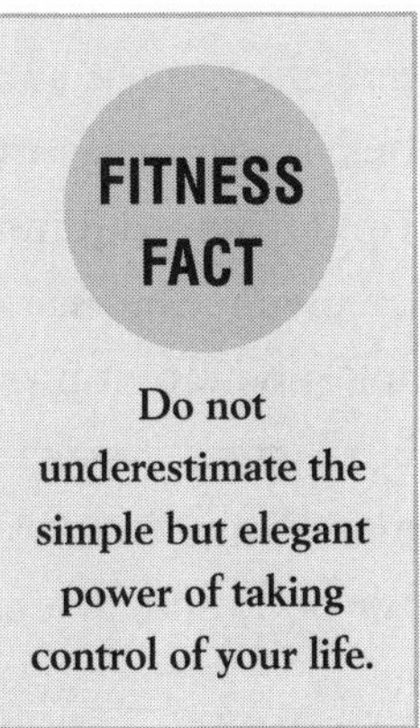

Mary is a thirty-five-year-old computer consultant who has learned techniques to manage stress and, as a result, seen improvements in her sex life. She runs an independent contracting business out of her apartment and therefore controls her own work schedule. She loves the flexibility of getting to choose whom she works with on what projects and when. But she often can't help herself, and accepts so many projects at once that she has to operate at maximum capacity. During these periods, Mary frequently works eighteen-hour days. She constantly feels stressed-out and behind schedule. She also finds that her sex drive disappears.

When Mary had a chance to relax, she used to spend an hour or two in front of the TV "spacing out." Recently, however, she realized that this was not enough to make her feel in control of her life. She felt that passively watching television wasn't doing her any good. She decided to take up a more involved and self-aware stress-reduction activity and devote time to it on a regular basis. Therefore, she began attending yoga classes three times a week at a gym near her house. She has also learned to meditate, and tries to practice this stress reduction technique every morning for fifteen minutes.

Mary now feels that she is taking control of her stress. She finds that she is more aware of her needs, emotions, and difficulties. Rather than shutting away the stress—and shutting down her sexuality at the same time—she instead makes an effort to embrace herself and her problems. She also finds that the enhanced self-awareness from yoga and meditation provides a "mental break" far superior to the one she used to get from television. Mary feels more relaxed and cheerful, more confident about herself and her capabilities, more in tune with her body and, as a result, says that she is more interested in and more likely to engage in sexual activity.

The following adjustments to lifestyle and attitude may require making substantial changes on your part, but they also yield the greatest rewards for the long term. Adapting your habits on an ongoing basis will better prepare you for dealing with all kinds of stress, from the everyday, mundane pressures of work to the less frequent but more severe anxiety created by illness or separation from a partner. Taking control of stress will make you feel better and, as a result, ensure that sexuality remains a regular, healthy part of your life.

1. Treat your body well.

The entire Sexual Fitness Program is based on the principle that what's good for your sexual health is good for you in general. If you eat well, sleep well, exercise, limit your use of medications, and make time to treat yourself to sensual activities, then you will relieve anxiety and tension as you optimize your sexual fitness. Studies show that maintaining healthy habits such as these helps reduce symptoms of and improve ability to cope with stress. When your body is in good physical condition and you feel positive about yourself, you are more competent in dealing with problems. You are naturally able to maintain a well-functioning cardiovascular system, boost hormone levels, control anxiety, and overcome other side effects of stress. You are therefore more likely to maintain a healthy interest in sex.

Value your body. You wouldn't allow your child to engage in harmful behaviors, so why should you allow yourself to? Treat yourself like the rare being that you are. Treasure your body because it's the only one you get—and it will reward you for this self-empowering and loving behavior.

2. Exercise regularly.

Exercise reduces stress. Repeated clinical trials reveal that people who are aerobically fit have less of a physiological response to and faster recovery from stress than do the unfit. Exercise improves your mood and takes your mind off your troubles by boosting levels of endorphins, chemicals in the brain that generate a sense of well-being. In your battle to combat stress, it's critical that you stay active.

In order to reap the maximum benefits of exercise, you do not always need to have a vigorous workout. You can enjoy cardiovascular benefits, keep your weight under control, and feel good about yourself as much from moderate-level exercise sessions (yoga, fast walking, golf, tennis) as from high-powered ones (running and biking long distances, aerobic workouts close to your maximum heart rate). What's more, there is no link between exercise intensity and mood. Stress levels drop by the same amount whether people engage in mild, moderate, or strenuous physical activity. So do what you love at a pace that you enjoy. Exercise is a time for you to clear your mind.

3. Include your kids in some of the activities you do.

If not spending enough time with your kids is one source of stress in your life—as it can be for many—and your schedule is tight, why not ask them to participate in some of these stress-relieving activities with you? After all, in this modern age children often have stress placed on them, as well. They have exams and papers for school, many compete in sports, others play instruments, and they may feel pressure to succeed. They can benefit from having you as a role model for how to handle the many demands of a busy life.

You can invite your kids to come with you on a walk, meditate with you, or even trade massages. You'll be helping yourself and your child, and as an added bonus you'll get to spend some high-quality time together.

At the same time, as we'll discuss next, it's also important to take a break from your kids. Taking care of them, their fighting, their homework demands, and so on mean that children are often a source of stress as well as a source of joy. Don't feel guilty about hiring a baby-sitter so that you can enjoy some much-needed time alone or with your partner on a regular basis.

4. Make time for your loved one.

While you may like to include your kids in some stress-reducing activities, it's still important that you have special time set aside just for you and your loved one. Yet with our stressful lives and busy schedules, this can be difficult to manage. Spontaneity is a myth. In order to ensure that you have relaxing, fun time together, the first step is to set up an appointment for romance about once a week. This tells your partner, "You are important to me." It reminds you both that your relationship is worth time and energy. While setting up regular dates may sound silly, it works for many couples.

You and your loved one could agree to "go out on a date," just as if you'd first met and were still in the early stages of courtship. This could be a weekly or a monthly event. But when the date night comes, there are no excuses. If you have kids, you may want to hire a baby-sitter or have your children stay the night with friends or family from time to time. You might even consider renting a hotel room for special occasions in order to get away from your usual surroundings and add some excitement and adventure to the evening.

There are different ways to spend time together. You and your partner can even have fun cleaning up the house or putting the kids to bed before you slip off for your time alone! Getting dressed can also be seductive and tantalizing. Wear an item of clothing that makes you feel sexy or a favorite sensual scent. You want to feel great about yourself. When it comes time for the date, take time to enjoy each other's company and really talk about what is going on in your lives. Then let events unfold naturally. Don't have any expectations that sex will occur: it may, it may not, and either way is okay.

5. Share your troubles.

Studies show that social support is one of the most effective methods of reducing stress. When you spend time with other people talking about your concerns, you not only gain perspective and insight, but your stress response actually slows. Take time to discuss your woes and concerns—as well as your good news—with your partner on a regular basis. The point is to maintain open communication, which will not only help you manage stress but also contribute to your trust, closeness, and understanding of each other. Aside from your partner, you might also talk with a family member, close friend, or co-worker. View-sharing is an opportunity for you to unburden yourself without leaving the problem up to the other person.

Regardless of whether or not you have a friend to talk to, you may also choose to see a mental health professional. Psychiatrists, psychologists, social workers, counselors, therapists, educators, and members of the clergy can all offer advice, teach life strategies, or simply lend an ear. Some people feel that therapy is too costly. But you would fix your car even when money is tight because you rely on it. Are your health and that of your relationship any less important? Other people may feel ashamed or embarrassed about seeking out professional counseling. But there is nothing shameful or embarrassing about dealing with the most important issues in your life. It takes courage to reach out for help. Don't hesitate to take advantage of this valuable resource. If you feel like it, then do it!

6. Enjoy the companionship of a pet.

Pets can also serve as excellent stress-reduction aids. They provide unconditional love, something that we all need and can't always count on getting from people. Pets are always there for you with a friendly lick or a loving purr. They also offer an opportunity for you to touch, cuddle, rub, and hug another being, which can be a source of immense comfort. Finally, pets give you something to care for and love. It's great to be needed.

Scientific research suggests that pets help to relieve stress, lower heart rate and blood pressure, speed recovery from illness, and improve general well-being. In a study of people treated for coronary heart disease, pet owners had a higher survival rate one year after hospital discharge than did nonowners.

7. Take daily breaks for what you enjoy.

Make sure to regularly take time out to enjoy yourself. And that doesn't mean just taking your annual vacation. Not everyone can save up fun or restful activities for special occasions every couple of weeks or even months. But experts say that you'll relieve stress more effectively by enjoying yourself every day than by rewarding yourself infrequently. Consistency is the key. You want to get into the habit of taking care of yourself. So take a break every day. Ensure that you have at least twenty minutes for your emotional needs alone. You could choose to spend your moment in the morning, at work, in the evening, even right before you fall asleep. Aside from these daily breaks, also be sure to take frequent mini-vacations. You might take an afternoon off from work or ask your family for a couple of hours one evening for yourself alone. Just make it happen.

As for what to do during your breaks, choose whatever makes you happy. Read, listen to music, soak in the bathtub, go fishing, bake a pie, or do whatever else strikes your fancy. Pay attention to the little things—eating your favorite fruit, reading the comics, or just watching the clouds drift by. Don't hesitate, don't compromise, and don't delay—do it now! You need it and you deserve it.

Remember, too, that when you are happy, when you feel good about yourself, and when you are treating yourself well, you are more likely to be interested in intimacy. You'll feel sexier, be more able to give of yourself, connect better with your partner, and more easily let go and enjoy the moment when you're engaged in sexual activity.

Don't wait for the two weeks a year when you literally get to "leave your worries behind." Even if only for a few minutes, go ahead and abandon them today. We have only a finite number of heartbeats—how are you going to use them?

Specific Stress-Reduction Techniques

In addition to incorporating some of the lifestyle strategies just discussed, which may require making real changes to the way you think and behave, there are specific actions you can take to make stress more manageable. Here is a list of stress-reduction techniques that you can pick up and start using today. They're easy to do, and none need be time-consuming. All of them should provide some level of immediate stress relief. They may also offer long-term benefits if you do them often enough.

In addition, many of these activities provide you with an opportunity to explore and appreciate your sensuality. Take the time to focus on how your body is responding to the exercises. Becoming self-aware should help to relieve stress as well as to stimulate your sexuality. Again, stress reduction is all about choice. You decide what to try, and you discover what works best for you. These activities are fun and pleasurable, so enjoy yourself!

1. Breathing

Breathing deeply and in a controlled fashion is the simplest, most effective technique for reducing stress. Without proper breathing, many of the other stress-reduction methods described here, including massage, visualization, and meditation, will be much less effective. What's more, breathing costs nothing and everyone can do it.

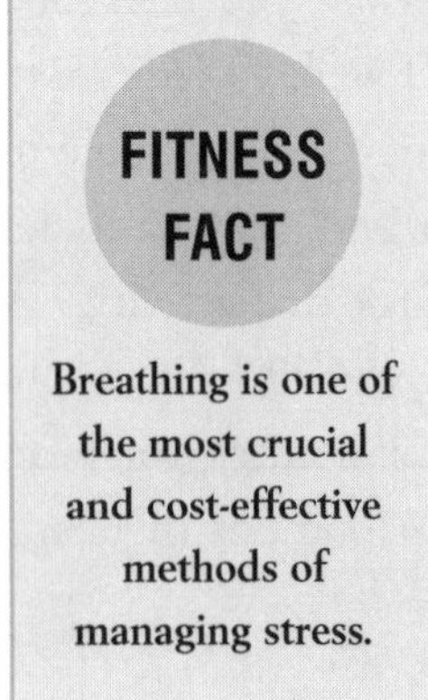

Breathing is one of the most crucial and cost-effective methods of managing stress.

When we become anxious, our bodies automatically react by stimulating a series of physiological responses including increased breathing rate. In preparation for fight or flight, we breathe shallowly, rapidly, and from the upper chest. Doing so might help us run faster, but it does not help us cope with stress.

In fact, this type of breathing will only serve to make you feel more tense and upset.

You can override this automatic response by learning to control your breathing. Proper breathing technique serves to increase oxygen flow, relax the body, and improve concentration. According to some practitioners, controlled breathing can also enhance sexual enjoyment. It is a cornerstone of Tantric sex (see chapter 4: *Sensual Stimulation*). Paying attention to your breathing leads to a general awakening and awareness of your body.

Below, you will find some breathing exercises to try. You'll be surprised at how quickly you can master these techniques with just a little practice and concentrated effort.

A. Deep breathing

Deep breathing counteracts the flight-or-fight response, forcing our bodies to slow down. This technique is best practiced on a regular basis, for about five minutes twice a day. If done at bedtime, it can help you fall asleep.

Lie down in a dark, quiet place like your bedroom. Close your eyes. Begin by simply noticing your breath. Pay attention as you inhale and exhale. Now take several slow, deep breaths, inhaling through the nose and exhaling through the mouth. Pull the air all the way into the bottom of your belly. You may want to place your hands on your stomach so that you can feel your abdomen contracting and expanding. Imagine the oxygen flowing through your entire body, filling your lungs and then traveling out to your fingertips and toes.

An advanced technique from yoga involves controlling your breath in a more focused manner. You may want to try this after you've mastered deep breathing. Take in one-third of your full breathing capacity, hold for three seconds, then exhale completely. Now take in one-half of your capacity, hold for three seconds, and exhale. Next take in two-thirds capacity, hold for three seconds, then exhale. Finally, take in full capacity, hold for three seconds, and exhale. Once you've completed this cycle, begin again.

B. Muscle relaxation

This technique is especially helpful if you carry your stress in the form of muscle tension. If you feel tight, your shoulders are cramped at the end of the day, and you just can't seem to loosen up, this technique is for you. It's also a great way to prepare yourself for sexual activity.

Lie down and close your eyes. Take a few calming breaths. Now imagine each of the muscles of your body relaxing, one by one. Begin with your head. Breathe in and observe the tension, even contract the muscle to identify it. Then let the breath out and release the tension along with it. Allow your eyebrows to relax, followed by the rest of your face, head, and neck. Move all the way through your shoulders, arms, hands, and fingers. Move next to your chest, abdomen, thighs, calves, and feet, then end with your toes. Imagine all your stress draining out of you. By the time you finish, you should feel like jelly—just a loose, comfortable mass of relaxed muscle.

C. Taking control

This breathing technique is particularly helpful for regaining a sense of control over yourself and your environment during stressful moments. It may prove helpful as part of a therapy program for people suffering from panic attacks.

Take a concentrated, deep breath every time you start to feel panicked—when you're stuck in traffic, when you hear your phone ring, when you look at your watch and realize that you're running late. Just one deep breath will help you focus on your ability to manage stress and remind you not to get so worked up. If you feel like it, you can even let out a sigh. Just sit back, say "Ahh," and feel your troubles drift away.

2. Meditation and yoga

In recent years, meditation has become a popular method of stress reduction. Meditation has been reported to lower blood pressure and heart rate, improving circulation by causing blood vessels to relax. It can also boost mood by stimulating the release of endorphins.

There are many different types of meditation, such as transcendental and mantra, vipassana and tara. Yoga is also a form of meditation that adds stretching and poses to deep breathing and clear thinking. It is practiced by the old and young alike. Some older people who do yoga feel that it helps them to retain their body height and posture.

Whichever type of meditation you choose, you should consider starting out in a class with an instructor who can guide you through the learning process. With yoga, it is crucial to begin with a class in order to avoid injury. Classes can be found at gyms and health clubs, yoga centers, and even some workplaces. For an extra boost to your sexual fitness, you might try couples yoga, which emphasizes poses involving two people. With an understanding of the basics and the assistance of an instructional book or videotape, you should later be able to practice meditation or yoga in your own home.

Below, you will find brief introductions to the practice of meditation and yoga. These are in no way intended to substitute for instruction by a trained professional.

Meditation Basics

1. Ensure a quiet environment where you can be for at least fifteen minutes without interruption.
2. Sit down on a pillow and cross your legs in front of you.
3. Rest your hands on your knees with the palms facing up.
4. Keep your back straight and your neck relaxed.
5. Close your eyes.

6. Take deep, even breaths. Focus on each one.
7. Try to clear your mind of all thoughts. You might want to repeat a particular word or sound over and over again—or buy a tape with these sounds. Suggestions include counting, making a simple sound such as "*mmm*," or saying "Peace," "It's okay," or some other calming phrase.
8. Relax this way for at least ten minutes a day.

Principles of Yoga

1. Avoid eating at least one hour prior to class.
2. Dress in loose, comfortable clothing. Shoes and socks will not be needed, as yoga is always practiced in bare feet.
3. You will need a sticky mat for the floor to prevent you from slipping. These are sometimes provided in class.
4. A yoga session generally focuses on three areas: breathing, meditation, and body postures.
5. You will generally begin with a warm-up and breathing exercises. Then you will move on to a series of postures, some that you may be familiar with and some that may be totally new. You should be given a chance to relax after every three to four movements.
6. The goal of the postures is to stretch various muscle groups. Never overextend yourself or make yourself feel uncomfortable.
7. Throughout these motions, you should continue to focus on your breathing.
8. You will probably end the session with a rest period or meditation. You should leave feeling relaxed and calm.
9. Practitioners stress that the more often you can practice yoga, even for short sessions, the better.

3. Visualization

Visualization offers many of the benefits provided by meditation. It can help decrease anxiety and take the body out of the stress mode. Women in labor may use visualization or self-hypnosis to help ease the anxiety and pain of childbirth. Athletes often use visualization to improve their technique and performance.

Visualization is easy to do, especially with practice. You can include imagery along with your meditation and breathing exercises: they are all complementary, and they all involve a few moments of peace.

Treat yourself to a mental vacation. Close your eyes. Imagine that you are in your favorite place on Earth. It may be a forest with gentle sunlight peeking through the leaves and birds chirping, a sunny beach with salty air and pounding surf, or a snow-covered mountaintop. You can also engage in more active visualization. For example, you can envision yourself flying through the air with the soft flutter of birds' wings around you, or swimming through the depths of the ocean surrounded by colorful fish. Wherever you go, it should make you feel calm and happy. You are limited only by your own imagination.

Carefully visualize yourself in this environment. Picture it down to the last little detail. Include all the senses. How does your skin feel? What are you wearing? Are there butterflies, fish, or birds to accompany you? What sounds do you hear? Do you walk around or sit still? You might encounter another person as you drift in this state. What does he or she have to say? As you enjoy your perfect space, feel your stress slip away. Continue for at least five to ten minutes—or for as long as you like.

Sex therapists often teach visualization techniques to women who have difficulty achieving orgasm. These women may find that they lose sensation and are unable to "let go" when they come close to having an orgasm. If they visualize what orgasm might feel like, what they would say or do if they achieved orgasm, then sometimes this projection allows them to lose conscious control. Reflex takes over the body from the mind. In this way, one may learn to achieve orgasm by imagining oneself through it.

4. Massage

Massage therapy truly is a magical treatment for the mind and body. It relaxes muscles, improves circulation, and induces a feeling of well-being. It has been reported to reduce blood pressure, relieve pain, enhance mental focus, and boost the immune system. It also offers an excellent way to relieve stress and stimulate sexual arousal.

Massage combats stress by telling the body that it is time to calm down, regardless of what the mind might be thinking. When your muscles experience pressure or kneading, they relax and muscular tension eases away. This sends chemical messages to your brain telling it that everything is okay. In other words, you mechanically force your body to halt the stress response. Levels of stress hormones fall. Your parasympathetic nervous system, the one responsible for relaxation and sexual arousal, kicks in. You feel more in tune with your body, more sensually aware, and more relaxed.

As we discussed in chapter 4: *Sensual Stimulation*, touch also works directly to reduce stress and enhance sexual pleasure by stimulating the release of oxytocin. If you remember, this hormone has a calming effect, lowers blood pressure, and encourages bonding behavior including sexual intimacy.

Massage need not be a long and involved process that adds to your overall stress level. Set easy-to-achieve goals for yourself, such as exchanging a five-minute massage with your partner once a week when you first climb into bed. You'll be amazed at how much of a difference these few minutes of physical connection with your lover can make in your life. (See the section on Touch in chapter 4: *Sensual Stimulation* for specific massage techniques).

5. Laughter

"Laughter is the best medicine," the saying goes. Well, it's true. How can you possibly feel tense when you're laughing? Laughter is the opposite of the stress response. It makes you feel happy, improves your mood, and helps you forget your troubles. Laughter also has a direct impact on stress by reducing muscle tension and blood pressure and lowering levels of stress hormones. And let's not forget that laughing just feels good.

So the next time you're having a tough day, try laughter therapy to make yourself feel better. Here are a few helpful laughing hints:

- Watch a tape of your favorite comedian or turn on the morning cartoons. There's nothing like a little Bugs Bunny to get you off to a good start.
- Spend more time with friends. According to researchers, when you're being social you're thirty times more likely to laugh. Laughter is contagious.
- Try something new. Take up dancing or pottery. You'll probably end up laughing at yourself during the learning process.
- Poke fun at yourself. Remember not to take your problems or your shortfalls too seriously.
- Make an effort to laugh. When you read a funny cartoon or hear a good joke, don't just chuckle silently to yourself. Instead, let out a really big guffaw. Chances are, you'll start those around you laughing as well.

6. Nature

There's real wisdom in the old saying "Take time to stop and smell the roses." Nature has a calming effect for many people. It reminds us that we are part of a bigger picture, that our problems are relatively insignificant. It also helps us remember not to move through life so quickly. Nature progresses gradually, in a slow, steady rhythm. It never rushes a new season to start or a flower to bloom. These are just a few of the reasons why it is so important to get outside. Go for walks and heartily breathe in the fresh air. Stroll along the beach and watch the waves roll in. Sit on a tree stump and listen to the forest. If you usually do your exercise outdoors, be sure to take some extra time just to appreciate your surroundings. Allow yourself to absorb the messages that nature is sending you.

If you can't be in nature on a regular basis, then surround yourself with reminders of the natural world at home and in the office. This can be particularly valuable if you live in a big city. Fill your rooms with plants. Bring fresh flowers home. Try to keep living things in your house all the time. The bright colors and pleasant aroma will cheer you up and calm you down. Also, you can enjoy the sounds of nature. There are literally hundreds of recordings of nature sounds available, from ocean waves to rainfall to birdsong. Try listening to these sounds when you are feeling tense, falling asleep, or meditating and relaxing. They offer a great antidote to stress.

7. Music

Anyone who regularly tunes in to music knows how soothing it can be. The gentle sounds and delicate rhythms, passionate melodies and familiar refrains help us to achieve a more relaxed frame of mind. Intuitively, we understand this. But a recent study of mood music put this commonsense notion about the calming powers of music to the test. Healthy adults listened to classical music by such famous composers as Debussy, Ravel, Bach, and Brahms while pondering their problems. After twelve weeks, all of them reported feeling less fatigue and depression and were in a better overall mood. Their levels of the stress hormone cortisol also fell significantly. What's more, the music continued to work its magic even after the study ended, reducing stress for at least seven weeks more.

Aside from the classical genre used in this experiment, any music that is simple, repetitive, and low pitched can effectively reduce stress. You might prefer New Age, monastic chants, folk songs, lullabies, love ballads, or easy-listening jazz. It's up to you.

So the next time you're looking for a little relaxation, put on that CD player, sit back, and have a listen. Or, if you feel like it, sing along! Singing aloud can also be a wonderful way to express yourself and relieve stress.

8. Aromatherapy

One way to help yourself relax is to enjoy the scents of nature. Aromatherapy is the art of using plant and flower essences for therapeutic purposes. Recall from chapter 4: *Sensual Stimulation* that aromatherapy is also a valuable method of stimulating your senses. It can make you aware of your body and awaken you to sexual desire.

Among other scents, aromatherapists recommend lavender and orange to alleviate tension. They often employ bergamot and chamomile fragrances to help relieve anger and irritability. Cedar and ylang ylang may be used to reduce anxiety.

You can practice aromatherapy in many different ways. Light a scented candle or burn incense. Buy fragrant flowers to decorate your home. Exchange massages with your partner using scented oils. Fill your bathtub with specially designed aromatherapy bath salts and oils. Buy an aromatherapy diffuser and allow the scent to waft through your home. Experiment with a variety of methods—just don't forget to breathe in and enjoy the calming aroma.

9. Warm water

Comfortably warm water has a remarkable ability to melt troubles away. Bathing relieves muscle tension, enhances circulation by dilating blood vessels, and can even improve your mood. Taking a hot bath before going to bed can also help you to achieve a deeper, more restful state of sleep. You can enjoy the stress-relieving qualities of warm water through a soak in a bathtub, hot tub, or natural hot springs, or even a stint in a steam room.

Bathing offers one of the easiest and most convenient forms of warm water relaxation. Set aside a block of time for your baths so that you can really relax. Close the door in order to shut yourself off—figuratively and literally—from the chaos of your life. Allow your mind to pleasantly wander. Remember to drink plenty of water, as the high temperature of the bathwater will likely cause you to sweat. Some people enjoy reading a novel or listening to music while bathing. If you choose to engage in another activity besides soaking, just be sure that it doesn't increase your stress level. After all, the goal is to "get away from it all," not to take it with you.

10. Herbal supplements

People have used plants, flowers, and herbs to treat physical and psychological problems for thousands of years. In fact, many modern medicines are made directly from plant materials. According to herbalists and traditional healers, there are several herbs that effectively combat stress, including chamomile, kava kava, and St. John's wort.

Chamomile, a European flower, is known for its mild soothing effects. It reportedly helps people feel calmer, and is typically used as a sleep aid. You can brew yourself some chamomile tea whenever you start to feel stressed-out or want to unwind before going to bed. Be aware that some people are allergic to chamomile. If you have allergic reactions to chrysanthemums, ragweed, or other flowers in the aster family, you should probably avoid this herb. Otherwise, chamomile is not known to have any side effects.

The kava kava plant offers another natural antistress treatment. The Polynesians drink a mixture of kava and coconut milk to induce a pleasant, somewhat euphoric state of being. In repeated clinical trials, kava has been proven a powerful tool for relieving anxiety. Unlike alcohol or other sedatives, kava kava is nonaddictive and has no unpleasant hangover effect. Take the recommended dose of capsules or tincture—about 60 to 120 mg per day. Or, for a delicious bedtime treat, mix up a batch of Kava Cocoa before you slip off to sleep (see the recipes section). Kava should not be taken in combination with any substances that act on the central nervous system, such as alcohol, barbiturates, or antianxiety and antidepressant medications.

St. John's wort, a flowering plant native to Europe, is a popular herb for boosting mood. In Germany, extract of St. John's wort is a more common treatment for depression than are prescription medications. Over ten years of clinical trials have demonstrated that St. John's wort is an effective antidepressant, elevating mood. It also has few side effects. The typical dose for treatment of depression is 300 mg of St. John's wort three times a day, and the herb takes about four weeks to have an effect. Do not take the herb if you are on any antidepressant medications.

Think Sexy, Be Sexy

The final component of stress reduction is having the right attitude. It's great to have confidence in your sexiness and believe in yourself. You *should* be proud of who you are and what you look like. Sexiness cannot exist without self-confidence, and sexual fitness depends not just on your physiological condition, but also on what you think of yourself—your attitude. In order to optimize your sexual satisfaction, it helps to believe that you are sexy. Here are some suggestions to help you feel great about yourself:

1. Make a list of all the things you like about yourself.

What are your favorite body parts? Your favorite facial features? What makes you different and beautiful? Now make a similar list of all the things you like about your partner. Once you have both made lists, share them with each other. Don't argue with your partner if he says that you have great hair and you disagree. Don't be shy when your lover compliments you on your beautiful smile. Just listen and accept the praise. Revel in it.

2. Spend time every day looking at yourself in the mirror.

Appreciate your mind and body, because together they make an incredible instrument. They allow you to be who you are. They give you pleasure. Thank your body for everything it does for you. Learn to adore it for all that it is, rather than disliking it for all that it isn't. The more you look at yourself, the more comfortable you will become with your body and your sexuality. Over time, you will grow to accept it and, more important, to love it.

3. Write down positive affirmations.

Spend some time writing down reaffirming statements about yourself, such as "I am sexy," "I inspire others," or "I have beautiful eyes." Carry these statements with you always, on cards in your wallet. Read them whenever you start to feel bad about yourself or your appearance. Use them to give yourself an ego boost. Remind yourself of why you're lucky to be you.

4. Throw out your fashion magazines.

Okay, that may be a bit extreme. But for women and a growing number of men, trendy magazines are a major source of angst about sexuality and appearance. These publications make it seem as though everyone is gorgeous and everyone is having fabulous sex all the time. They may make you feel that your body and your looks aren't good enough. Nothing could be further from the truth. You do not need to compare yourself with these unrealistic standards. Avoid them. Set your own standards for yourself and your loved ones—everyone has unique characteristics that they should treasure!

You're Ready to Make Yourself Sexually Fit!

You've done it! You've taken the first step toward optimizing your sexual passion, pleasure, and satisfaction by reading this book. You've gained the basic knowledge needed to take control of your sexual vitality. In the first three chapters, we discussed how changing your eating habits, nutrition, and medication use will turn your body into a more efficient sex machine. In these past four chapters, we've discussed a number of techniques you can use to further enhance your sexual fitness and the overall quality of your life. Sensual stimulation will help you discover whole new realms of pleasure, exercise will get you in the proper physical and mental shape for peak performance, sleep and stress reduction will ensure that you have energy for and interest in sexual activity in the first place.

Now it's time for you to put this newfound knowledge to work for you, and to develop positive habits that will last a lifetime. The Sexual Fitness Program offers a comprehensive, day-by-day guide to reaching your full sexual potential over the next thirty days.

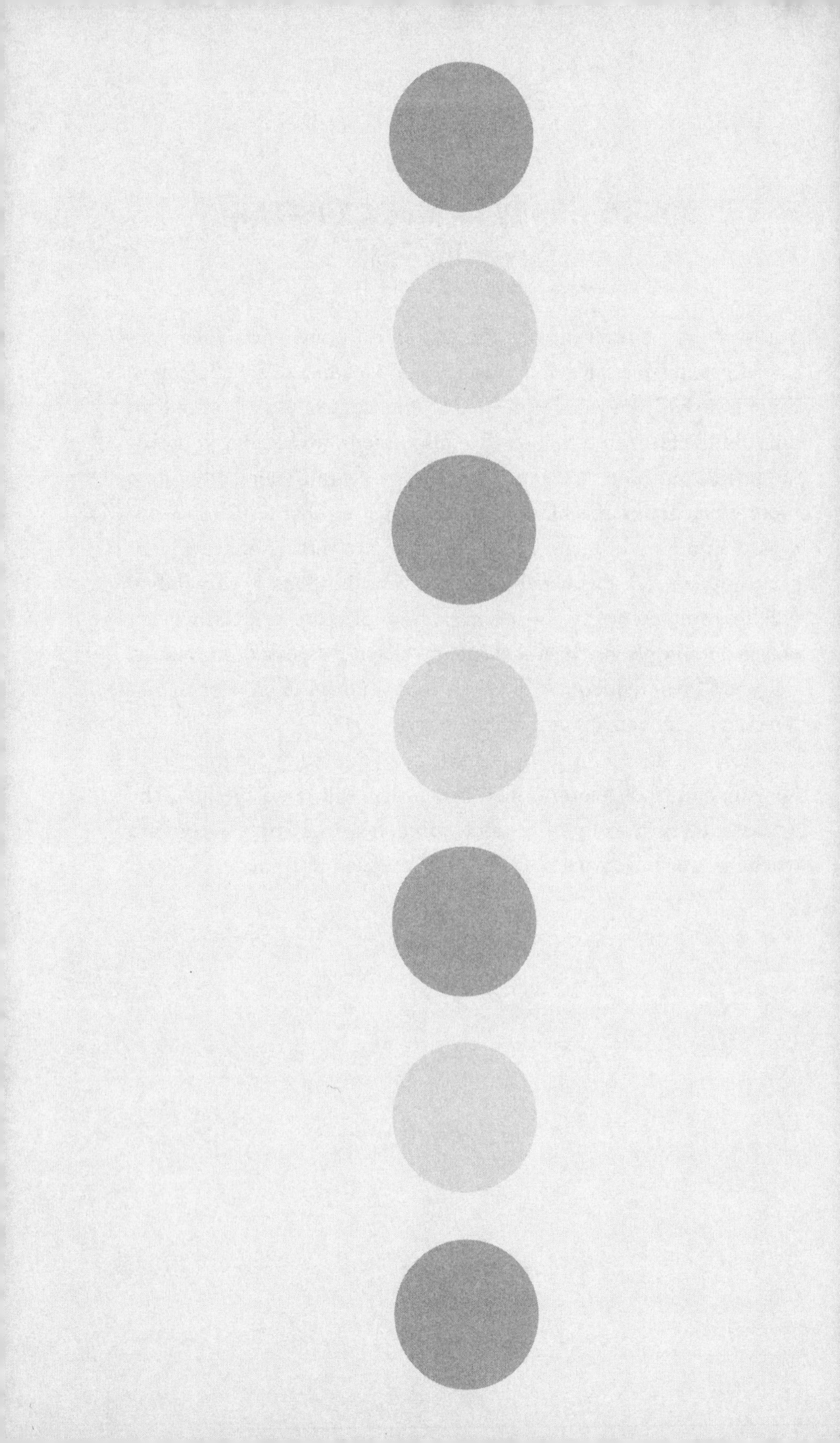

The 30-Day Sexual Fitness Program

The 30-Day Sexual Fitness Program is outlined below in an easy-to-follow format. Every day, you will find headings for each of the seven essential elements leading to sexual fitness: Diet, Supplements, Medications, Sensual Stimulation, Sleep, Stress Reduction and Exercise.

Under the Diet category, you're provided with a daily meal plan and recipes for most items. You can follow the meal plan exactly, mix items around, or make substitutions with similar foods. For example, feel free to swap dinners and lunches, repeat your favorite recipes more often, include some of your own healthy recipes, or substitute chicken for tofu. Certain recipes (when noted) in the program often yield enough food to last more than one meal. These can make great leftovers if you like, and you can use them for a lunch or dinner suggested later in the week. Desserts are definitely optional.

Note that the program begins on a Saturday. This is due to the fact that activities listed for Saturdays and Sundays tend to be more involved, with the assumption that you have more free time and energy on weekends. If this is not the case, rotate your schedule so that the days marked "Saturday" and "Sunday" correspond with your weekends, whenever they may fall.

You'll be asked to keep a record of what you do every day and how it affects your sexual passion, pleasure, and health. Writing down what you do on a daily basis will motivate you to stick with the program and remind you of your accomplishments. Check boxes are provided next to each item, so that once you've completed the activity or eaten the food you can check off the box. If you don't do it, make a note to yourself about why. Jot down your thoughts and ideas. Make the program interactive.

In fact, we'd love to know what works for you! We welcome your comments, questions, and suggestions online. Would you like to ask about specific activities and recommendations, learn about the latest health research, share a new recipe with other people on the Sexual Fitness Program, or tell others about your experiences? Would you like to get customized feedback on your progress? Visit our Web site: **www.sexualfitnessMD.com** for information, support, and interaction with others in the sexual fitness community.

DAY 1

Saturday: Preparation Day

1. DIET: Remind yourself of the Six Nutritional Steps to Sexual Fitness:

1. Cut back the fat.
2. Reduce cholesterol.
3. Munch on more fruits and vegetables.
4. Eat whole grains, nuts, and seeds.
5. Add more soy to your diet.
6. Spice up your life.

Be sure to drink at least eight 8-ounce glasses of water today and every day of the program. Begin by cleaning out your cupboards and refrigerator. Throw away all the foods that you'll want to avoid now that you're on the Sexual Fitness Program: If they're not easily available to you, then you're less likely to eat them. Here is a list of foods to toss—or at least consume in minimal amounts.

Foods to Minimize

- Butter, margarine, and shortening
- Whole dairy products: whole milk, cream, half-and-half, ice cream
- Regular-fat cheese
- Coconut and palm oils
- Mayonnaise
- Fatty cuts of meat; chicken and turkey with skin
- Fried foods

- Packaged baked goods, candies, and crackers
- Packaged meat products (e.g., hot dogs, hamburgers, luncheon meats)
- Any packaged foods high in fat (e.g., macaroni and cheese, certain frozen meals, soups made with cream base)
- Processed grains: white bread, refined pasta

2. SUPPLEMENTS: First, check with your doctor to ensure that you can take these supplements, as you would before initiating any new nutritional plan. Refer to chapter 2 for charts listing all the ingredients of the supplement plans for male and female sexual fitness.

Once you get medical clearance, purchase the recommended supplements, either individually or as a preformulated product, and begin taking them today (optional). You might also purchase the herbs separately, and get the recommended vitamins and minerals from a multivitamin.

3. MEDICATIONS: Schedule an appointment with your doctor to discuss the potential impact of any prescription medications that you take regularly. Write down the date of your appointment here:

____

Make a list of all the medications you take on a regular basis here. Bring it with you to your appointment.

1. ____________________	4. ____________________
2. ____________________	5. ____________________
3. ____________________	6. ____________________

You may want to ask your doctor for a full physical evaluation. You could be suffering from a health problem that is interfering with your ability to enjoy sex. Ask your doctor to investigate any health concerns that might be having an impact on your overall wellness and sexual fitness, including checking hormone levels.

4. SENSUAL STIMULATION: Purchase, or pick out from your collection, several CDs of music that you and your partner find sensual, romantic, or simply enjoy listening to when you're relaxing. Listen to at least one of them today while you're relaxing, cuddling with your partner, or getting ready for bed. Write down the names of a few of your favorite albums here:

1. ______________________	4. ______________________
2. ______________________	5. ______________________
3. ______________________	6. ______________________

5. EXERCISE: If you're not already physically active on a regular basis, then make an exercise plan for yourself today. Begin walking, join a gym in your neighborhood, sign up for fitness classes, buy exercise videos, or get a commitment from a friend or your partner to work out with you. Do what it takes to make sure that you will make exercise a part of your routine at least four days a week. Make it happen TODAY!

6. SLEEP: Check if your bedroom is quiet and comfortable enough to be conducive to optimal sleep by asking yourself the following questions:

1. Are your pillow and mattress comfortable? If not, you may need to buy a new pillow, a mattress that has more support, or perhaps a "feather bed" to cover your current mattress. Do you have any allergies? Consider purchasing products made from allergy-free materials.
2. Does noise wake you up during the night or early in the morning? If so, consider purchasing a white noise machine or earplugs.

3. Does sunlight wake you up in the morning? If so, you may need to get better blinds or hang heavier material over your windows. Or purchase a mask to wear over your eyes in the morning.
4. Is the room temperature comfortable throughout the night? If not, perhaps you need to buy an air conditioner, space heater, or fan.

Make a list of things you need to buy based on your answers to these questions.

7. STRESS REDUCTION: Spend some time thinking about the effect that stress has on your life. Do you feel in control of what's going on around you most of the time? Do you wish that you had more time to yourself? Would you like to get better at managing stress? Write down your thoughts and steps you'd like to take to manage stress better here: ____

____

____

EXTRA: Fill out the Sexual Fitness Survey provided in the *Introduction*. Keep it in a safe place so that you can compare your answers with those you get at the end of the program.

DAY 2

Sunday: Preparation Day

1. DIET: Go shopping! Fill your home with foods that you want to eat because they're fresh and appealing, but will also make you feel good. Here is a shopping list:

Fresh Foods:

• Fruits: oranges, grapefruits, bananas, grapes, peaches, pineapples, apples, apricots, tomatoes, figs, dried fruits of any kind, and whatever else looks good.

• Vegetables: leafy greens like spinach, kale, collard greens, dandelion greens, and chard; broccoli, asparagus, artichokes, lettuce, cucumbers, and whatever else looks appealing. Choose frozen over canned vegetables if fresh produce is not available.

• Whole grains, nuts, and seeds: brown and wild rice; whole-grain pasta, whole-grain bread, whole-wheat flour, oats, and barley; peanuts, cashews, almonds, walnuts; sesame seeds, etc.

• Protein: tofu, fish, oysters, skinless chicken and turkey with all fat removed, extra-lean cuts of other meats for special occasions, nonfat dairy products such as cottage cheese, yogurt, and milk; beans.

Herbs and Spices:

• Cumin, curry, cayenne pepper, chili peppers; fresh herbs like basil, dill, oregano, rosemary, and parsley; garlic and ginger.

Prepackaged Foods:

- Natural, low-fat packaged dinners
- Veggie burgers
- Soy products
- All-natural, low-fat pasta sauces, salad dressings, and marinades
- All-natural, nonfat sorbets and fruit bars for dessert

2. SUPPLEMENTS: Take the recommended supplements (optional).

3. MEDICATIONS: Use the following chart to start recording what medications you are currently taking and to keep track of the side effects, if any. This is a good way to get in touch with what you are putting into your body and to be proactive with your health.

	TAKING	SIDE EFFECT
Antihypertensives		
Antidepressants		
Anti-ulcer drugs		
Cold/Allergy medications		
Hormones		
Prosexual drugs		
Other		

Also, every day for the rest of the program, record the amount of cigarettes, caffeine, and alcohol that you consume. Performing this activity will help remind you not to have more than the recommended daily amount of these substances.

4. SENSUAL STIMULATION: While you're out grocery shopping today, pick out a variety of items with interesting, sensuous, or stimulating smells. For example, you might purchase cinnamon sticks and vanilla beans, licorice candies, fresh cherries and strawberries. You might even bake chocolate chip cookies or a pumpkin pie. Later in the day, try a Scent Experiment with your partner. Breathe in deeply of each item to fully experience the smell. Note here how each one makes you feel. Do any of the scents turn you on, make you feel sexy, or remind you of a favorite sexual experience?

Item: ____________________ Feelings: ____________________
Item: ____________________ Feelings: ____________________
Item: ____________________ Feelings: ____________________
Item: ____________________ Feelings: ____________________

5. EXERCISE: Do at least thirty minutes of a cardiovascular activity such as walking, swimming, biking, or playing tennis or basketball. If you're a beginner, work at least a half hour of physical activity into your routine in the form of "lifestyle exercise" (e.g., park at the far end of the parking lot, walk up stairs, rake leaves). Write down what you did and for how long, today and every day for the rest of the program.

Activity: ______________________________

Length of time: ______________________________

6. SLEEP: Buy any of the products (listed yesterday) that you need to help you sleep better: earplugs, blinds, new pillow or mattress, fan, etc. Record your sleep patterns today and every day for the entire program. Rate your estimated general energy level throughout the day on a scale of 1 to 5, with 1 being very low and 5 being very high.

Time to bed: ______ Time awake: ______ Energy level: ______

7. STRESS REDUCTION: Read through the notes you wrote down yesterday about stress. Based on this list, pick one stress-management activity and try it today.

DAY 3

Monday

1. DIET: Prepare the following meals in accordance with the guidelines presented in the overview of this chapter. Do the same every day for the rest of the program. Recipes are included for all menu selections marked with an asterisk (*). Desserts are always optional. At the end of the day, make notes about which recipes you liked best. Also record how closely you followed the meal plans and any substitutions that you made—what you actually ate.

	MEAL PLAN	WHAT I ATE / NOTES
Breakfast	Ginger Mango Shake* or Quick Oatmeal*	
Lunch	Miso Soup* Tofu-Spinach Pizza Rolls*	
Dinner	Dijon-Style Tempeh* Savory Wild Rice* Steamed Fresh Broccoli	
Dessert/ Snack	Cheesecake Mousse with Raspberry Sauce*	

2. SUPPLEMENTS: Did you remember to ask your doctor if it's okay for you to take the supplements? If so, start taking them today (optional).

3. MEDICATIONS: Continue recording what medications you are currently taking and keeping track of the side effects, if any.

	TAKING	SIDE EFFECT
Antihypertensives		
Antidepressants		
Anti-ulcer drugs		
Cold/Allergy medications		
Hormones		

	TAKING	SIDE EFFECT
Prosexual drugs		
Other		

4. SENSUAL STIMULATION: Look at the list you made yesterday of stimulating scents. Purchase a variety of items with these scents to keep around the house. For example, you might buy aromatherapy candles, bath oils, perfumes, or colognes that are based on your favorite smells. Now you'll have them available anytime you feel like stimulating your senses, creating a romantic mood, or adding a new "scent-ual" dimension to your lovemaking.

5. EXERCISE: If you are just beginning to exercise and are therefore concentrating on lifestyle exercise, then do at least thirty minutes of physical activity today. If you are already engaged in at least a moderate level of exercise, you can take the day off (optional).

Activity: ______________________________

Length of time: ______________________________

6. SLEEP: Set up your room with your new purchases to ensure an optimum sleep environment. If your energy level yesterday and today was low, try to get more sleep tonight.

Time to bed: ______ Time awake: ______ Energy level: ______

7. STRESS REDUCTION: One of the key components in managing stress and enjoying your sexuality is feeling good about yourself. Look at yourself in the mirror and think about your favorite attributes. What do you like about yourself? What are your favorite body parts? What are your favorite personality traits? Write them down so that you can read this list as a reminder to feel really positive about yourself.

____

Concentrate on appreciating who you are—with all your special and unique characteristics. Congratulate yourself on what you've done to improve your sexual fitness today!

DAY 4

Tuesday

1. DIET: Prepare the following meals.

	MEAL PLAN	WHAT I ATE / NOTES
Breakfast	Banana Latte* or Whole-Grain Cereal*	
Lunch	Asian Cabbage Salad* Dijon-Style Tempeh*	
Dinner	Fiery Fish Fillets* Steamed Brown Rice* Easy Asparagus*	
Dessert/ Snack	Kava Kava Cocoa*	

2. SUPPLEMENTS: If you've received approval from your physician, take the recommended supplements (optional).

3. MEDICATIONS:

	TAKING	SIDE EFFECT
Antihypertensives		
Antidepressants		
Anti-ulcer drugs		
Cold/Allergy medications		
Hormones		
Prosexual drugs		
Other		

If you drink caffeine regularly, consuming more than mild to moderate amounts every day may be interfering with your sexual fitness. Moderate use is defined as 200 to 300 mg per day: about two cups of coffee or four cans of soda.

4. SENSUAL STIMULATION: Tonight when you and your partner climb into bed, or perhaps in the morning when you awake, or even for a noon break if you prefer, spend at least five minutes just kissing. Explore the sensation of feeling each other's mouths and bodies pressed together. Do not worry about expectations of further sexual activity. Instead, concentrate only on your sensations in that instant. Remember what it felt like when you first started dating? Relax and enjoy.

5. EXERCISE: Do at least thirty minutes of a cardiovascular activity such as walking, swimming, biking, playing tennis, golfing, or gardening.

Beginners can continue to work at least a half hour of physical activity into your routine in the form of "lifestyle exercise."

Activity: ___________________________________

Length of time: ______________________________

6. SLEEP: If you have trouble falling asleep at night, try drinking a glass of warm milk or chamomile tea, taking a bath just before you go to bed, or establishing another calming bedtime ritual. Did performing this activity help you out? Make notes tomorrow morning:

____

____

____

Time to bed: ______ Time awake: ______ Energy level: ______

7. STRESS REDUCTION: Try the "take control" breathing exercise described in chapter 7. Take a deep breath and exhale loudly every time you notice yourself feeling stressed. Remember that you can use this quick, simple, and cost-free method to relieve stress anytime, any day of the week. You can also take a few deep breaths when you climb into bed at night in order to help yourself fall asleep. Breathe.

DAY 5

Wednesday

1. DIET: Prepare the following meals.

	MEAL PLAN	WHAT I ATE / NOTES
Breakfast	Blueberry Smoothie* or Whole-Wheat Toast	

	MEAL PLAN	WHAT I ATE / NOTES
Lunch	Spring Salad with Avocado and Shrimp*	
Dinner	Vegetarian Chili* Whole-Wheat French Bread Fresh Green Salad	
Dessert/ Snack	Blackberry Crisp*	

2. SUPPLEMENTS: Take the recommended supplements (optional).

3. MEDICATIONS:

	TAKING	SIDE EFFECT
Antihypertensives		
Antidepressants		
Anti-ulcer drugs		
Cold/Allergy medications		
Hormones		
Prosexual drugs		
Other		

Heavy alcohol consumption interferes with sexual performance. If you drink alcohol, you should try to drink no more than two glasses in a single day.

4. SENSUAL STIMULATION: Light some candles either during dinner with your partner or in the bedroom when you're ready to retire for the evening. Enjoy the sensual nature of the soft lighting. In addition, make a list of sensual activities, such as massage, listening to music, or kissing that you most enjoy prior to lovemaking. Encourage your partner to do the same. Share these lists with each other and make a commitment to do more of them over the coming weeks.

____

____

____

____

5. EXERCISE: If you are just beginning to exercise and are therefore concentrating on lifestyle exercise, then do at least thirty minutes of physical activity today. If you are already engaged in at least a moderate level of exercise, you can take the day off (optional).

Activity: ______________________________________

Length of time: _________________________________

6. SLEEP: Remember that exercising late in the evening can interfere with sleep. Try to get your exercise in earlier in the day.

Did the activity you tried yesterday to help you fall asleep work? If not, you might consider taking a *natural* sleep aid, such as melatonin or valerian, just before you're ready to go to bed.

Time to bed: ______ Time awake: ______ Energy level: ______

7. STRESS REDUCTION: Determine how and when you'd like to practice meditation or yoga. Find out if there are classes you can take at your gym, office, or in your neighborhood. Consider purchasing a "how-to" video or book. Take the initial steps to make meditation possible for you.

Schedule a "date night" with your partner for Saturday. Plan ahead on this one—don't wait until the last minute.

DAY 6

Thursday

1. DIET: Prepare the following meals.

	MEAL PLAN	WHAT I ATE / NOTES
Breakfast	Pineapple-Peach Smoothie* or Fruit Plate	
Lunch	Chinese Chicken Salad* Vegetarian Chili*	
Dinner	Soybean-Vegetable Minestrone* Spinach and Mushroom Manicotti* Fresh Green Salad*	
Dessert/ Snack	Chocolate Almond Tapioca Pudding*	

2. SUPPLEMENTS: Take the recommended supplements (optional). If you have not yet started the supplement program but have your doctor's approval, you may want to consider beginning it now. For many people, it has a noticeable impact on energy levels and sexual satisfaction.

3. MEDICATIONS:

	TAKING	SIDE EFFECT
Antihypertensives		
Antidepressants		

	TAKING	SIDE EFFECT
Anti-ulcer drugs		
Cold/Allergy medications		
Hormones		
Prosexual drugs		
Other		

4. SENSUAL STIMULATION: Practice nonsexual touch for at least ten minutes. As you're getting ready for bed, take a warm shower. Then dim the lights, put on some soft music, and perhaps light a few candles in the bedroom. Now cuddle, hug, kiss, and caress your partner. Try not to have any expectations that further sexual activity will occur. Just enjoy the physical sensations your body experiences. How did this exercise make you feel?

____

____

____

5. EXERCISE: Continue to do at least thirty minutes of a cardiovascular activity such as walking, swimming, biking, playing tennis, golfing, or gardening. Beginners can continue to work at least a half hour of physical activity into your routine in the form of "lifestyle exercise."

Activity: ________________________

Length of time: ____________________

6. SLEEP: If you do drink coffee or smoke, be sure not to consume either, or any other stimulants, after 6 P.M. Keep this up for the duration of the program.

Time to bed: ______ Time awake: ______ Energy level: ______

7. STRESS REDUCTION: Have you been keeping up with the stress-reduction activities that you committed to at the beginning of the program? If so, congratulations. If not, it is never too late to get started! Remember that stress has a powerful ability to destroy sexual interest and enjoyment.

DAY 7

Friday

1. DIET: Prepare the following meals.

	MEAL PLAN	WHAT I ATE / NOTES
Breakfast	Mixed Fruit Smoothie* or Quick Oatmeal*	
Lunch	Soybean-Vegetable Minestrone* Whole-Wheat French Bread	
Dinner	Mussels with Vermicelli* Fennel Salad with Herbal Dressing*	
Dessert/ Snack	Peach-Blackberry Stew*	

2. SUPPLEMENTS: Take the recommended supplements (optional).

3. MEDICATIONS:

	TAKING	SIDE EFFECT
Antihypertensives		
Antidepressants		
Anti-ulcer drugs		
Cold/Allergy medications		
Hormones		
Prosexual drugs		
Other		

4. SENSUAL STIMULATION: If you engage in sexual activity today, encourage your partner and allow yourself to make noise during lovemaking. Feel free to express yourself vocally. Enjoy sighing, moaning, screaming, or letting escape whatever other sounds come naturally to you.

5. EXERCISE: Feel free to take the day off if you've been regularly keeping up with the exercise program (optional). Congratulate yourself on a job well done!

Activity: ______________________________

Length of time: ______________________________

6. SLEEP: Do not consume alcohol in order to fall asleep, and avoid it after 10 P.M. Although it is a relaxant, alcohol increases the incidence of nighttime awakenings.

Are you enjoying your new bedroom setup? Are you sleeping

better as a result? Have you been keeping up your calming nighttime ritual?

Notes: ____

____

Time to bed: _____ Time awake: _____ Energy level: _____

7. STRESS REDUCTION: Try a short visualization exercise today for at least ten minutes. Lie down in a quiet room and close your eyes. As you breathe deeply, clear your mind of all thoughts and concerns. Now imagine being in your ideal place, a place that makes you feel happy and relaxed. Visualize all the details, from how the air feels and smells, to the sounds you hear. Describe that ideal here:

____

____

____

DAY 8

Saturday: Date Night

1. DIET: Prepare the following meals or enjoy a healthy but sensuous dinner out. Be sure to drink at least eight glasses of water today and every day!

	MEAL PLAN	WHAT I ATE / NOTES
Breakfast	Very Berry Smoothie* or Whole-Grain Cereal	
Lunch	Spinach Salad with Tofu Dressing* Vegetarian Chili*	

	MEAL PLAN	WHAT I ATE / NOTES
Dinner	Sizzling Tandoori Shrimp* Basmati or Brown Rice Cucumber Salad	
Dessert/ Snack	Sensuous Strawberry Peach Kabobs*	

2. SUPPLEMENTS: Take the recommended supplements (optional).

3. MEDICATIONS:

	TAKING	SIDE EFFECT
Antihypertensives		
Antidepressants		
Anti-ulcer drugs		
Cold/Allergy medications		
Hormones		
Prosexual drugs		
Other		

When dining out or celebrating, it can be difficult to control your drinking, smoking, and caffeine consumption. However, the goal of the program is to enjoy satisfying sexual experiences and overdoing it with any of these substances will only take away from your sexual performance and pleasure.

4. SENSUAL STIMULATION: Tonight during your "date" with your partner, enjoy each other's company without feeling any sense of urgency or expectation. Dress so that you feel sexy. Have fun and be flirtatious. Take it slowly. Savor every sensation. Perhaps you might like to try some of the activities you wrote down earlier in the program of favorite sensual stimulation exercises? How did you do? __________

____

____

____

5. EXERCISE: It's the weekend, so try to push yourself a bit harder on your exercise routine. If you usually work out for thirty minutes, try going for forty. If you usually do forty-five minutes of exercise, boost it up to sixty. If you usually walk, run, or swim, pick up your pace a bit. In the end, you should feel a little more invigorated than you normally do. Challenge yourself. Good job!

Activity: ______________________________________

Length of time: _________________________________

6. SLEEP: Many people tend to stay up much later and sleep in longer on the weekends. However, this can upset your sleep schedule. If you can, stick roughly to your routine times for going to bed and waking up even on Saturdays and Sundays. You might like to stay up and sleep in an hour or two longer, but try to avoid altering your schedule much more than that. You'll feel more alert and prepared to deal with the world, both over the weekend and all the next week, if you do.

Time to bed: ______ Time awake: ______ Energy level: ______

7. STRESS REDUCTION: Tonight is date night, which means that you and your partner agree to take the night off just for each other. Go out for a romantic dinner or relax and prepare your meal together. Don't have any particular agenda, sexual or otherwise, as this can only contribute to your stress. Instead, just focus your efforts on having fun and enjoying each other's company.

DAY 9

Sunday: Outdoors Day

1. DIET: Prepare the following meals. If the weather cooperates, pack your pasta lunch as a picnic and take it along on your outdoor adventure.

	MEAL PLAN	WHAT I ATE / NOTES
Breakfast	Breakfast Milkshake* or Whole-Wheat Toast	
Lunch	Penne Pasta with Mediterranean Vegetables* Whole-Grain Bread	
Dinner	Indian Chicken Curry* Basmati or Brown Rice	
Dessert/ Snack	Cheesecake Mousse with Raspberry Sauce*	

2. SUPPLEMENTS: Take the recommended supplements (optional). Are you keeping up with your supplements on a daily basis? Keep it up!

3. MEDICATIONS:

	TAKING	SIDE EFFECT
Antihypertensives		
Antidepressants		
Anti-ulcer drugs		
Cold/Allergy medications		
Hormones		
Prosexual drugs		
Other		

4. SENSUAL STIMULATION: Sometime today, buy flowers that are beautiful and smell fragrant. Bring them home and arrange them in a vase or in several places around the house. They will scent your rooms with natural smells, remind you of the outdoors, and bring happy thoughts to mind all week.

5. EXERCISE: If the weather is decent, skip your usual routine to enjoy a long, relaxing walk outdoors today. Go to a park if you live in a city, or if you're in the countryside already then go someplace new. If you regularly walk or run for exercise, don't follow your usual path. Discover a new area to explore. If the weather prevents you from being outside, then at least do a new activity that's different from your normal exercise habit.

Time spent walking/hiking: ______________________________

6. SLEEP: After your outdoor exercise, you should sleep soundly. Remember, today and throughout the rest of the program, not to eat

or drink too much just before you go to bed. You want to avoid upsetting your stomach or waking up frequently during the night to use the bathroom.

Time to bed: ______ Time awake: ______ Energy level: ______

7. STRESS REDUCTION: Nature has a marvelous ability to remind us that our problems are not really so bad, relieve our stress, and boost our spirits. So when you are outside today, take a few extra moments to revel in your surroundings. Breathe deeply. Enjoy the fresh scents and clean air. Take time to look around you and appreciate the natural beauty of the world.

DAY 10

Monday

1. DIET: Are you sticking at least roughly to the meal plans? Have you reduced your consumption of red meat, high-fat foods, packaged baked goods, and other items on the taboo list? Are you remembering to eat plenty of fresh fruits, vegetables, and whole grains? If you slipped, don't give up! Try again. Each day makes a difference. Each week you'll improve. You can do it!

	MEAL PLAN	WHAT I ATE / NOTES
Breakfast	Ginger Mango Shake* or Fruit Plate	
Lunch	Noodle Salad with Toasted Sesame Dressing* Easy Asparagus*	

	MEAL PLAN	WHAT I ATE / NOTES
Dinner	Broccoli-Stuffed Potatoes* Fresh Green Salad	
Dessert/ Snack	Strawberry Rhubarb Cobbler*	

2. SUPPLEMENTS: Take the recommended supplements (optional).

3. MEDICATIONS:

	TAKING	SIDE EFFECT
Antihypertensives		
Antidepressants		
Anti-ulcer drugs		
Cold/Allergy medications		
Hormones		
Prosexual drugs		
Other		

4. SENSUAL STIMULATION: Tonight, enjoy the scents of one of the items you recently purchased—light an aromatherapy candle, bathe in a scented tub, or burn some incense. Did it make you feel sexy? Record what you did and how it made you feel:

____

____

____

5. EXERCISE: By now you should be getting used to your workout routine. As you can see, exercise is recommended at least four days a week in this program—Saturdays, Sundays, Tuesdays, and Thursdays. Monday is optional. And remember that if you're incorporating physical activity regularly into your life through less structured "lifestyle exercises" (e.g., walking the dog, gardening), you need to do at least thirty minutes of this every day.

Activity: ____

Length of time: ____

6. SLEEP: How are you sleeping? Is your bedroom environment as conducive to sound sleep as it should be? Do you still feel comfortable with your pillow and mattress, noise level, light exposure, and temperature throughout the night? If not, go back to Day 1, read through the questions, and make the necessary changes now. You're worth it.

Time to bed: ______ Time awake: ______ Energy level: ______

7. STRESS REDUCTION: Spend at least five minutes today laughing. Call up an old friend whom you used to laugh with, listen to a tape of your favorite comedian, watch some cartoons, read the comic strips in the paper, or see a funny movie. Laugh out loud; don't hold back—make it count, and make it a habit.

DAY 11

Tuesday

You are now one-third of your way through the Sexual Fitness Program. This is a good time to check on your status. Review the progress you've made so far by reading through your notes and looking at your journal entries. Have you been keeping up? If so, take a moment today to look at yourself in the mirror and congratulate yourself. If you've been having some difficulties, don't worry. You can improve today! Start exercising, work on one eating habit that you'd like to change, see your doctor for advice on quitting smoking, or do something else that makes you feel that you've made a difference. Remember, you have the power to control your sexual passion, pleasure, and health. You can do it!

1. DIET: Don't forget that writing down what you eat every day will help you to stay focused and motivated.

	MEAL PLAN	WHAT I ATE / NOTES
Breakfast	Banana Latte* or Quick Oatmeal*	
Lunch	Herbed Chicken, Potato, and Olive Salad* Fresh Fruit	
Dinner	Grilled Salmon* Steamed Red Potatoes Curried Greens*	
Dessert/ Snack	Grape Sorbet*	

2. SUPPLEMENTS: Take the recommended supplements (optional).

3. MEDICATIONS:

	TAKING	SIDE EFFECT
Antihypertensives		
Antidepressants		

	TAKING	SIDE EFFECT
Anti-ulcer drugs		
Cold/Allergy medications		
Hormones		
Prosexual drugs		
Other		

Have you seen your doctor to talk about the medications you're taking?

4. SENSUAL STIMULATION: Trade massages with your partner for about ten minutes this evening before you go to bed. If you like, you can use massage oil scented with one of your favorite smells. For suggestions of how to give and receive a massage, review the charts in chapter 4.

5. EXERCISE: Continue to do at least thirty minutes of a cardiovascular activity such as walking, swimming, biking, playing tennis, golfing, or gardening. Beginners can continue to work at least a half hour of physical activity into your routine in the form of "lifestyle exercise."

Activity: ______________________________

Length of time: ______________________________

6. SLEEP: Are your feet warm enough at night? Try wearing socks to bed and see if that helps you fall asleep more easily. Also, don't forget to try taking a warm bath, drinking tea or warm milk, or listening to calming music just before you go to bed.

Time to bed: ______ Time awake: ______ Energy level: ______

7. STRESS REDUCTION: Lie down in a quiet, comfortable place where are you ensured privacy for a short time. Try the deep breathing exercise described in chapter 7 for at least fifteen minutes. Feel the air fill your lungs and belly, then exhale slowly. Also, remember to practice "take control" breathing throughout the day by taking deep breaths whenever you feel a wave of anxiety or tension rising within you.

DAY 12

Wednesday

1. DIET: It's easy to go completely off the meal plan part of the program simply because you slipped for one or two days. Don't let this happen to you. Instead of feeling guilty and giving up, just get right back into it as soon as possible. Remember, any change at all is better than none.

	MEAL PLAN	WHAT I ATE / NOTES
Breakfast	Blueberry Smoothie* or Whole-Grain Cereal	
Lunch	Great Green Quiche* Fertility Booster Fruit Salad*	
Dinner	Nutty Brown Rice and Spinach Casserole* Steamed Fresh Broccoli	
Dessert/ Snack	Peach-Blackberry Stew*	

2. SUPPLEMENTS: Take the recommended supplements (optional).

3. MEDICATIONS:

	TAKING	SIDE EFFECT
Antihypertensives		
Antidepressants		
Anti-ulcer drugs		
Cold/Allergy medications		
Hormones		
Prosexual drugs		
Other		

4. SENSUAL STIMULATION: Buy some chocolate sauce, whipped cream, ice cream, or honey. Place a large towel on the floor and ask your partner to lie down. Now spread some toppings on your lover and then eat them off! Depending on how you think your partner will react, you may want to discuss this with him or her first or make it a surprise. What do you think? ______________________________

____

____

____

5. EXERCISE: Unless you are doing "lifestyle exercise," in which case you need to keep up with thirty minutes a day, you can have the day off if you wish. Spend some of your time and energy today on learning meditation or yoga instead.

Activity: ____

Length of time: ____

6. SLEEP: Do you take naps? If so, have you been alert and energetic during the day? Remember that napping can prevent you from sleeping soundly through the night. But if a brief snooze helps you make it through a long day, just remember to limit your naps to no longer than thirty minutes.

Time to bed: ______ Time awake: ______ Energy level: ______

7. STRESS REDUCTION: Have you thought about looking for a meditation or yoga center in your neighborhood, found an instructor, or ordered a video or book? If so, learn to practice yoga or meditation for thirty minutes today.

Plan for a "date night" with your partner for Saturday. Think ahead as to how you'd like to spend the evening. Make dinner reservations or arrange for a baby-sitter if necessary.

DAY 13

Thursday

1. DIET: Are you noticing a difference in your energy level because of your healthy diet? Remember not to overeat. Eat only when you are hungry, and stop eating as soon as you feel full. Take your meals slowly.

	MEAL PLAN	WHAT I ATE / NOTES
Breakfast	Pineapple-Peach Smoothie* or Whole-Wheat Toast	

	MEAL PLAN	WHAT I ATE / NOTES
Lunch	Health Nut Burgers* Green Salad	
Dinner	Scallop Sauté on Steamed Swiss Chard* Whole-Grain French Bread	
Dessert/ Snack	Kava Kava Cocoa*	

2. SUPPLEMENTS: Take the recommended supplements (optional).

3. MEDICATIONS:

	TAKING	SIDE EFFECT
Antihypertensives		
Antidepressants		
Anti-ulcer drugs		
Cold/Allergy medications		
Hormones		
Prosexual drugs		
Other		

4. SENSUAL STIMULATION: Wear a new perfume or cologne. Pay close attention to how your partner reacts when you first see him or her in the evening. Then ask your lover to evaluate the scent. What does he or she think?

Also, find the name of a salon that offers massage therapy or an individual masseur or masseuse online or in the yellow pages—or, even better, get a recommendation from a friend. Book an appointment for a professional massage for you and your partner for Saturday.

5. EXERCISE: You're really making exercise a part of your daily life. The longer you keep it up, the better you will feel, and the more likely you are to make it a regular habit. Stick to it!

Activity: ______________________________

Length of time: ______________________________

6. SLEEP: You should be getting at least six hours of sleep every night. Are you? Did the chamomile tea or Kava Kava Cocoa you drank today help you fall asleep?

Time to bed: ______ Time awake: ______ Energy level: ______

7. STRESS REDUCTION: Prepare some chamomile tea or Kava Kava Cocoa. Drink at least one cup with your partner just before going to bed.

DAY 14

Friday

1. DIET: With parties, trips to restaurants, and family events going on, it can be difficult to keep up good eating habits over the weekend. Remember to stay focused on your goal of a better sex life and improved overall health.

	MEAL PLAN	WHAT I ATE / NOTES
Breakfast	Mixed Fruit Smoothie* or Fruit Plate	
Lunch	Ratatouille* Whole-Grain French Bread	
Dinner	Pizza Primavera* Fresh Spinach Salad	
Dessert/ Snack	Chocolate Almond Tapioca*	

2. SUPPLEMENTS: Take the recommended supplements (optional).

3. MEDICATIONS:

	TAKING	SIDE EFFECT
Antihypertensives		
Antidepressants		
Anti-ulcer drugs		
Cold/Allergy medications		
Hormones		
Prosexual drugs		
Other		

4. SENSUAL STIMULATION: Listen to one of your favorite romantic-music albums for at least twenty minutes at the end of the day. Do so either while relaxing alone or while cuddling with your partner so that you really listen. Dim the lights. Let the music wash over you. Feel how it affects your mood.

5. EXERCISE: If you're engaging in regular, structured exercise at least four times a week, use this day to relax and prepare for the weekend if you like. Keep up the "lifestyle exercise" if this is your routine.

Activity: ____

Length of time: ____

6. SLEEP: Have a good night's sleep. Remember not to throw off your regular schedule by going to bed or waking up much later than usual.

Time to bed: ______ Time awake: ______ Energy level: ______

7. STRESS REDUCTION: Take a break today to do one of your favorite relaxation activities, which you listed at the beginning of the program. Read a book, play with your pet, walk barefoot on the grass, talk with an old friend, or eat an ice-cream cone. Do something just for you.

Activity: ____

DAY 15

Saturday: Date Night

Congratulations! You are halfway through the 30-Day Sexual Fitness Program. Take this day to reward yourself for all your amazing accomplishments, your dedication, motivation, and progress so far. You should already be noticing a difference in your energy level and overall health, your sense of self-empowerment, and perhaps even in your sexual interest and pleasure. But you can keep improving, so don't stop now!

1. DIET: Enjoy these sensuous and seductive meals or treat yourself to dinner out at a restaurant.

	MEAL PLAN	WHAT I ATE / NOTES
Breakfast	Very Berry Smoothie* or Quick Oatmeal*	
Lunch	Garden Fresh Pasta* Whole-Grain Bread	
Dinner	Roasted Red Pepper Soup* Scalloped Oysters* Easy Asparagus*	
Dessert/ Snack	Blackberry Crisp*	

2. SUPPLEMENTS: Are the supplements you're taking making a difference? If so, continue to take them consistently. If not, don't give up. Nutritional supplements can take up to one month to have a noticeable effect on some people. It's not too late to start the supplement program if you haven't done so yet.

3. MEDICATIONS:

	TAKING	SIDE EFFECT
Antihypertensives		
Antidepressants		
Anti-ulcer drugs		
Cold/Allergy medications		

	TAKING	SIDE EFFECT
Hormones		
Prosexual drugs		
Other		

You can treat yourself to a glass or two of wine or beer with dinner. It's a celebration, after all!

4. SENSUAL STIMULATION: Treat yourself and your partner to a fabulous professional massage. You're worth it! Although it's enjoyable and pleasurable to exchange massages with each other, a professional can work on problem areas and teach you new techniques. Be sure to arrive a few minutes early so that you're relaxed for your appointment. Afterwards, spend some more time relaxing (sauna, steam room, hot tub, or warm shower if available would be great) rather than rushing on to the rest of your day.

5. EXERCISE: If you've been doing "lifestyle exercise" for the past two weeks, it's time to take your activity level up a notch. Start participating in regular, structured exercise at least four times a week. If you haven't yet joined a gym, signed up for an exercise class, or agreed to work out with a friend, then take this opportunity to do so. Make your commitment to an active lifestyle concrete. Do cardiovascular exercise for at last thirty minutes today.

Activity: ______________________________

Length of time: ______________________________

6. SLEEP: Massage helps improve the quality of your sleep. You should sleep soundly tonight!

Time to bed: ______ Time awake: ______ Energy level: ______

7. STRESS REDUCTION: It's date night! Take this evening to spend some high-quality time with your partner. Make sure that you can enjoy each other's company at a leisurely pace. You should have already enjoyed a sensuous massage today. Now connect by holding hands and breathing deeply together, with eyes closed or open, depending on which you prefer. Feel the flow of positive energy from one of you to the other.

DAY 16

Sunday: Day for Changes

1. DIET: Buy a food that you've never tried before today: soybeans or soymilk, wheat germ or some other grain, an exotic vegetable or fruit. Experiment! Also, remember to keep drinking water every day. It's a critical component of a healthy diet.

	MEAL PLAN	WHAT I ATE / NOTES
Breakfast	Breakfast Milkshake* or Whole-Grain Cereal	
Lunch	Red Pepper Soup* Your New Food Whole-Grain Bread	
Dinner	Crab Enchiladas* Spanish Rice Fresh Green Salad	
Dessert/ Snack	Grape Sorbet*	

2. SUPPLEMENTS: Take the recommended supplements (optional).

3. MEDICATIONS:

	TAKING	SIDE EFFECT
Antihypertensives		
Antidepressants		
Anti-ulcer drugs		
Cold/Allergy medications		
Hormones		
Prosexual drugs		
Other		

4. SENSUAL STIMULATION: Many couples complain that they lack sexual interest because they're tired of the same sexual routines. Here's something different: Make love in a new place. You might try sex in a new room of the house or even someplace slightly daring like outside in the backyard (make sure the neighbors can't see you—it's not fair to impose your sexual activity on an unwilling audience). Discuss this with your partner in advance. Trying something new will make you feel daring and bold, which can only serve to stimulate your sex drive. Also, taking risks together helps to build bonding and trust.

5. EXERCISE: There's no better way to stay motivated to exercise than to try new things. You don't want to get stuck in the same old routine day after day and slowly lose interest. So do something different today. If you usually run, then swim. If you usually golf, then play tennis instead. If you always work out at the gym, then do an outdoor workout today. Or try something completely new, like salsa lessons or in-line skating. Shake it up!

Activity: ______________________________

Length of time: ______________________________

6. SLEEP: When it comes to sleep, on the other hand, the best rule is not to make any changes. Try to stick to a routine sleep schedule.

Time to bed: ______ Time awake: ______ Energy level: ______

7. STRESS REDUCTION: If you've skipped any of the suggested stress-reduction activities so far, from breathing to meditation, make today your day to try one. No excuses! There's no reason not to try. If you don't like the activity, then don't do it again. If you do like it, then you've discovered a new and exciting way to enrich your life.

New activity: ______________________________

DAY 17

Monday

1. DIET: Are you feeling good about the new eating patterns you're establishing? Don't look at the program as a "deprivation diet," but rather as a change in lifestyle. If you learn to love the tasty and tantalizing foods recommended here, you're more likely to keep up these healthy habits after the program ends and for the rest of your life!

	MEAL PLAN	WHAT I ATE / NOTES
Breakfast	Ginger Mango Shake* or Whole-Wheat Toast	
Lunch	Spring Salad with Avocado and Shrimp* Whole-Grain Bread	
Dinner	Garden Fresh Stew* Brown Rice	
Dessert/ Snack	Apricot Fruit Chutney with Vanilla Nut Whip*	

2. SUPPLEMENTS: Take the recommended supplements (optional).

3. MEDICATIONS:

	TAKING	SIDE EFFECT
Antihypertensives		
Antidepressants		
Anti-ulcer drugs		
Cold/Allergy medications		
Hormones		
Prosexual drugs		
Other		

4. SENSUAL STIMULATION: Try an eye-contact exercise with your partner. While you are making love, keep your eyes open and focused on each other. How does this make you feel? Does it enhance your intimacy? Does it make you feel more connected? Have you revisited your and your partner's lists of favorite sensual stimulation activities? If not, now is the time. Perhaps you'd like to edit your lists based on the activities you've most enjoyed over the past few weeks on the Sexual Fitness Program.

____

____

____

____

5. EXERCISE: Are you committed to working out at least four times a week? Exercise is optional today if you've been sticking to this schedule. Good job!

Activity: ________________________________

Length of time: ___________________________

6. SLEEP: It's tempting to skimp on sleep when you get busy. Remember to make sleep a priority: it keeps you healthy, helps you manage stress, and improves your mood.

Time to bed: ______ Time awake: ______ Energy level: ______

7. STRESS REDUCTION: Try the muscle relaxation breathing exercise described in chapter 7. Inhale deeply. As you exhale, release the tension from a specific muscle group. Gradually work your way through your entire body. Remember also to take deep breaths anytime you feel stressed or anxious today and every day.

DAY 18

Tuesday

1. DIET: Make a note of your three favorite meals so far, or send us your own sexual fitness recipe and look for great new ideas online!

	MEAL PLAN	WHAT I ATE / NOTES
Breakfast	Banana Latte* or Fruit Plate	
Lunch	Fabulous Fresh Gazpacho* Green Salad	
Dinner	Shrimp Skillet with Orzo* Curried Greens*	
Dessert/ Snack	Cheesecake Mousse with Raspberry Sauce*	

2. SUPPLEMENTS: Take the recommended supplements (optional).

3. MEDICATIONS:

	TAKING	SIDE EFFECT
Antihypertensives		
Antidepressants		
Anti-ulcer drugs		

	TAKING	SIDE EFFECT
Cold/Allergy medications		
Hormones		
Prosexual drugs		
Other		

4. SENSUAL STIMULATION: If you're feeling adventuresome tonight, try this trick for enhancing oral sex. Munch on a mint or ice cube, or fill your mouth with a mint-flavored liqueur before beginning the activity. It should stimulate your partner by creating a tingling sensation in the genital region.

5. EXERCISE: How did you like that new activity you tried on Sunday? If you found it enjoyable and stimulating, then do it again! Try not to fall back into your usual routine. Participate in at least thirty minutes of cardiovascular exercise today.

Activity: ____

Length of time: ______________________________________

6. SLEEP: Remember that breathing exercises such as the one you tried yesterday are also effective methods for helping you fall asleep. Take a few deep breaths when you go to bed tonight.

Time to bed: ______ Time awake: ______ Energy level: ______

7. STRESS REDUCTION: Try a visualization exercise when you have at least ten minutes of calm and quiet today. Lie down in a dark room and take deep breaths for several minutes. Now begin to imagine your ideal sexual experience. How are you dressed? What does your partner look like? Where are you? What do your surroundings look and feel like? What do you do? How does it feel? Describe here:

____

____

____

____

DAY 19

Wednesday

1. DIET: Take a moment to congratulate yourself today. You're doing a great job so far!

	MEAL PLAN	WHAT I ATE / NOTES
Breakfast	Blueberry Smoothie* or Quick Oatmeal*	
Lunch	Miso Soup* Tuna Salad or Vegetable Sandwich	
Dinner	Island Chicken with Pineapple Salsa* Basmati or Brown Rice Steamed Fresh Broccoli	
Dessert/ Snack	Strawberry Rhubarb Cobbler*	

2. SUPPLEMENTS: Take the recommended supplements (optional).

3. MEDICATIONS:

	TAKING	SIDE EFFECT
Antihypertensives		
Antidepressants		
Anti-ulcer drugs		
Cold/Allergy medications		
Hormones		
Prosexual drugs		
Other		

If you're a regular coffee drinker, try to have decaf today.

4. SENSUAL STIMULATION: Step into your bedroom about five minutes before you retire for the evening. Light an aromatherapy candle or incense (in one of your favorite scents) then shut the door. When you enter the room a few minutes later, it should be filled with the wonderful, stimulating smell that you love so much. Take gentle breaths and enjoy the aroma.

5. EXERCISE: If you've been dedicated to your exercise program, you can take the day off today if you like.

Activity: ______________________________

Length of time: ______________________________

6. SLEEP: Are you still sleeping comfortably? Are there any changes you'd like to make to your bedroom? If there are, do so today.

Time to bed: ______ Time awake: ______ Energy level: ______

7. STRESS REDUCTION: By now you should have found an instructor or video and tried yoga or meditation at least once. The more you do it, the better you'll get and the more you'll be able to enjoy the results. So keep it up! Practice yoga or meditate for at least thirty minutes today.

Plan a "date night" for Saturday with your partner. Remember that being spontaneous may not always work. It's best to set aside time for each other.

DAY 20

Thursday

1. DIET: Don't forget to keep recording what you eat every day. And no cheating! Be honest with yourself—you'll do a better job of adapting your habits and embracing the new ones if you are.

	MEAL PLAN	WHAT I ATE / NOTES
Breakfast	Pineapple-Peach Smoothie* or Whole-Grain Cereal	
Lunch	Fennel Salad with Herbal Dressing* Fabulous Fresh Gazpacho*	
Dinner	Pasta with Green Sauce* Whole-Wheat French Bread Fresh Spinach Salad	
Dessert/Snack	Peach-Blackberry Stew*	

2. SUPPLEMENTS: Take the recommended supplements (optional).

3. MEDICATIONS:

	TAKING	SIDE EFFECT
Antihypertensives		
Antidepressants		
Anti-ulcer drugs		
Cold/Allergy medications		
Hormones		
Prosexual drugs		
Other		

4. SENSUAL STIMULATION: Trade foot massages with your partner. If you've never done or had one of these before, then you're in for a treat. Touch to the foot is incredibly pleasurable and even arousing for many people. Turn off the lights in the bedroom and light a few candles. Put on some soft mood music. Now enjoy rubbing and kneading each other's feet. Use a peppermint-scented foot lotion, which is both stimulating to the feet and arousing to the senses. Don't worry about this being a major time commitment—the massages need last only five minutes—but do put your love and care into it.

5. EXERCISE: You have been physically active for nearly three weeks now. How does it feel? Are you proud of yourself? You should be! Do at least thirty minutes of cardiovascular activity today.

Activity: ______________________________

Length of time: ______________________________

6. SLEEP: A stress-reducing foot massage should lead you into a restful night of sleep. Are you enjoying your bedtime routine of a cup of decaf tea, a glass of warm milk, a hot bath, or some other calming activity?

Time to bed: ______ Time awake: ______ Energy level: ______

7. STRESS REDUCTION: Make a list of all the things in your life for which you are grateful. Think about the items on the list carefully, considering how each one makes you feel. This exercise should help you escape from your daily problems and focus on the bigger, more important issues in your life. Do it whenever you feel particularly overwhelmed.

What I'm Grateful For: ______________________________

____

____

____

____

DAY 21

Friday

1. DIET: Get ready for the weekend, which can be full of temptations. Reinforce what you've learned already about the importance of nutrition by rereading chapter 1, if need be. Stay focused on your goal of enhanced sexual fitness!

	MEAL PLAN	WHAT I ATE / NOTES
Breakfast	Mixed Fruit Smoothie* or Whole-Wheat Toast	

	MEAL PLAN	WHAT I ATE / NOTES
Lunch	Asian Green Bean Salad* Grilled Vegetable, Tuna, or Tofu Sandwich	
Dinner	Dijon-Style Tempeh* Savory Wild Rice* Steamed Fresh Brocolli	
Dessert/ Snack	Apple Crisp (see Blackberry Crisp)*	

2. SUPPLEMENTS: Are you sticking to your supplement regimen? Remember that they're only effective if you take them consistently—that means every day. Take the recommended supplements (optional).

3. MEDICATIONS:

	TAKING	SIDE EFFECT
Antihypertensives		
Antidepressants		
Anti-ulcer drugs		
Cold/Allergy medications		
Hormones		
Prosexual drugs		
Other		

It's been three weeks! By now you should be noticing a difference in your sexual interest and pleasure.

4. SENSUAL STIMULATION: Pick out one of your favorite CDs from the collection you made at the beginning of the program. Play it when you are getting into bed or while you're taking your bath. Lie quietly and listen to the arousing sounds for several minutes while doing nothing else.

5. EXERCISE: Cardiovascular exercise is optional today if you've been following the program. Take the day off if you like.

Activity: ____

Length of time: ______________________________________

6. SLEEP: The quality of your sleep should be improving over the course of the program as you relax and exercise more, eat better, and devote time to yourself. Have you noticed a change? ____________

____

Time to bed: ______ Time awake: ______ Energy level: ______

7. STRESS REDUCTION: When you have guaranteed at least ten minutes of peaceful time, take the phone off the hook and draw yourself a warm bath. You may want to add scented bath oil. Turn off the lights and light a candle. Climb into the bathtub and soak. Feel your troubles melt away.

Return to the evaluation of stress in your life that you wrote at the beginning of the program. Have you effectively reduced stress? Do you feel more in control? If not, have you considered seeking out a counselor or therapist to talk to? Don't be shy or embarrassed to make use of this valuable resource.

____

____

DAY 22

Saturday: Date Night

1. DIET: It's date night! That means you should try to enjoy a sensuous meal with your partner, either at home or at a restaurant.

	MEAL PLAN	WHAT I ATE / NOTES
Breakfast	Very Berry Smoothie* or Fruit Plate	
Lunch	Asian Cabbage Salad* Dijon-Style Tempeh	
Dinner	Mussels with Vermicelli* Easy Asparagus* Whole-Wheat Bread	
Dessert/ Snack	Sensuous Strawberry and Peach Kabobs*	

2. SUPPLEMENTS: Take the recommended supplements (optional).

3. MEDICATIONS:

	TAKING	SIDE EFFECT
Antihypertensives		
Antidepressants		
Anti-ulcer drugs		
Cold/Allergy medications		

	TAKING	SIDE EFFECT
Hormones		
Prosexual drugs		
Other		

4. SENSUAL STIMULATION: Rent a sexy movie to watch with your partner during your date. Ensure that you will not be interrupted for at least a couple of hours. Turn down the lights, put on some comfortable clothes or your favorite lingerie/underwear, and lie down in a private place. Turn on the movie. Keep an open mind and allow yourself to become aroused when things get steamy. See where the spirit takes you.

5. EXERCISE: Do your best to take a companion along with you for your workout today. Consider engaging in physical activity with a best friend, your partner, a pet, or your children. Use this as an opportunity to exercise and to bond with someone whom you feel you never get enough time with.

Activity: ______________________________

Length of time: ______________________________

6. SLEEP: Try to keep to your usual weekday sleep schedule as much as possible.

Time to bed: ______ Time awake: ______ Energy level: ______

7. STRESS REDUCTION: Because it's date night, you're setting aside time specifically for you. You're investing in yourself and your relationship. What could be more worthy of your time and energy? Don't cheat yourself of this precious time together. During your date, remind your partner of why you think he or she is sexy. Talk about all your lover's favorite qualities. Then have your partner do the same for you.

DAY 23

Sunday: House Day

1. DIET: Are you remembering not to keep foods that you want to avoid around the house? If you don't have unhealthy snacks readily available in your kitchen cupboards, then you're far less likely to eat them.

	MEAL PLAN	WHAT I ATE / NOTES
Breakfast	Breakfast Milkshake* or Quick Oatmeal*	
Lunch	Ratatouille* Whole-Grain French Bread	
Dinner	Broccoli-Stuffed Potatoes* Spinach Salad with Tofu Dressing*	
Dessert/ Snack	Chocolate Almond Tapioca Pudding*	

2. SUPPLEMENTS: Take the recommended supplements (optional).

3. MEDICATIONS:

	TAKING	SIDE EFFECT
Antihypertensives		
Antidepressants		

	TAKING	SIDE EFFECT
Anti-ulcer drugs		
Cold/Allergy medications		
Hormones		
Prosexual drugs		
Other		

4. SENSUAL STIMULATION: What you see in your bedroom and how you feel about it helps determine how sensual and sexy you feel in it. If your bedroom is a tantalizing and arousing place, then you are more likely to become tantalized and aroused when you're there. Maybe you want to change the color of your bedroom or rearrange the furniture to make it into your ideal love nest. First, think of your ideal sexual experience, recorded earlier after a visualization exercise (Day 18). Then try to incorporate some of the elements into your room. Paint the walls, put up cloth hangings, buy more pillows for the bed, adjust the lighting, move the bed to a new location—do whatever it takes to make you and your partner feel that your bedroom is someplace special.

5. EXERCISE: Take a break from your work around the house to get out and exercise. Challenge yourself by pushing yourself beyond your usual routine. Exercise fifteen to thirty minutes longer than normal or try to complete your activity in less time. Make yourself work harder and you'll feel great afterwards.

Activity: ______________________________

Length of time: ______________________________

Also, think of an activity that you've always wanted to try—skydiving, horseback riding, scuba diving, surfing, ballet, skiing, in-line skating, kickboxing, belly dancing—something new and adventuresome. Look it up in the yellow pages or on the Internet, or get a recommendation from a friend, and figure out where you can try it. Book an appointment for next Sunday—you deserve it!

6. SLEEP: As you work on creating your ideal love nest, keep in mind that your bedroom should be sacred—for sleep and sex alone. You should not watch TV, pay bills, work, or do any other stressful activities there that will interfere with your ability to relax and enjoy sexual pleasure or sleep. So, clear out your desk, TV, and VCR. Get rid of those boxes and piles of paper that have accumulated over the years. Put up a divider if you don't have space to move everything to another room. Otherwise, get it out. Make your bedroom just that—a bedroom.

Time to bed: ______ Time awake: ______ Energy level: ______

7. STRESS REDUCTION: If you've rearranged your bedroom environment, then it's been a busy day! But it's worthwhile—in the end, your bedroom will be a much more pleasant place. Let it be a sanctuary for you. Keep your stress out of the room on a regular basis, so that you can retire there whenever you need a moment of peace. Create positive associations for yourself among your bedroom, sensual pleasure, and relaxation.

DAY 24

Monday

1. DIET: Remember, water is a critical component of a nutritious diet. Be sure to drink at least eight glasses of water today.

	MEAL PLAN	WHAT I ATE / NOTES
Breakfast	Ginger Mango Shake* or Whole-Grain Cereal	
Lunch	Herbed Chicken, Potato, and Olive Salad* Fresh Fruit	
Dinner	Grilled Salmon* Nutty Brown Rice and Spinach Casserole*	
Dessert/ Snack	Grape Sorbet*	

2. SUPPLEMENTS: Take the recommended supplements (optional).

3. MEDICATIONS:

	TAKING	SIDE EFFECT
Antihypertensives		
Antidepressants		
Anti-ulcer drugs		

	TAKING	SIDE EFFECT
Cold/Allergy medications		
Hormones		
Prosexual drugs		
Other		

4. SENSUAL STIMULATION: This evening try something new in bed. Agree with your partner in advance that you're going to talk to each other while you're engaged in sexual activity—and not just regular pillow talk, but some sexy, stimulating talk. Tell your partner exactly what it is that he or she does that most drives you wild. Or, if you feel comfortable, describe a sexual fantasy. Be explicit.

5. EXERCISE: You've been doing an excellent job. Take the day off if you worked out this weekend and at least four days last week.

Activity: ______________________________

Length of time: ______________________________

6. SLEEP: How do you like your new bedroom setup? Does it make you feel more calm and relaxed? Do you think you'll be able to drift off into slumber more easily now?

Time to bed: ______ Time awake: ______ Energy level: ______

7. STRESS REDUCTION: Have you been taking deep breaths whenever you feel anxious? Continue to practice "take control" breathing at particularly tense moments. Because you've been doing breathing exercises for a while now, you're ready for one that's more advanced. Spend at least fifteen minutes tonight doing the yoga breathing technique described in chapter 7 under "Deep breathing."

DAY 25

Tuesday

1. DIET: Skip one treat that you find really, really tempting today. Then congratulate yourself for sticking to the program.

	MEAL PLAN	WHAT I ATE / NOTES
Breakfast	Banana Latte* or Whole-Wheat Toast	
Lunch	Health Nut Burgers* Green Salad	
Dinner	Fiery Fish Fillets* Steamed Broccoli Whole-Wheat French Bread	
Dessert/ Snack	Strawberry Rhubarb Cobbler*	

2. SUPPLEMENTS: Take the recommended supplements (optional).

3. MEDICATIONS:

	TAKING	SIDE EFFECT
Antihypertensives		
Antidepressants		
Anti-ulcer drugs		
Cold/Allergy medications		

	TAKING	SIDE EFFECT
Hormones		
Prosexual drugs		
Other		

If you spoke with your doctor and made changes to your medications because of sexual side effects, have you noticed a difference?

4. SENSUAL STIMULATION: Take some time tonight to enjoy a few quiet moments alone. Shut the door and lie down on a bed surrounded by aromatherapy candles or slip into a warm bath. Revel fully in at least one of your senses. Appreciate how much your body has to offer you.

5. EXERCISE: Are you feeling the benefits of your new exercise program? Are you becoming addicted to the high of a great workout? Do at least thirty minutes of a cardiovascular activity today. If you're feeling bored with your exercise routine, try something new.

Activity: ______________________________

Length of time: ______________________________

6. SLEEP: If you're still feeling tired during the day, then increase your average sleeping time by at least thirty minutes.

Time to bed: ______ Time awake: ______ Energy level: ______

7. STRESS REDUCTION: "Laughter is the best medicine." Make sure that you have at least one hearty laugh today. Look up jokes on the Internet, read the comics, or engage in some pleasant banter with your partner or a colleague. Allow yourself to laugh heartily.

DAY 26

Wednesday

1. DIET: You have made a real commitment to long-lasting sexual and general health. You should feel proud of yourself!

	MEAL PLAN	WHAT I ATE / NOTES
Breakfast	Blueberry Smoothie* or Whole-Grain Cereal	
Lunch	Soybean-Vegetable Minestrone* Fertility Booster Fruit Salad*	
Dinner	Spinach and Mushroom Manicotti* Fennel Salad with Herbal Dressing* Whole-Wheat Rolls	
Dessert/ Snack	Blackberry Crisp*	

2. SUPPLEMENTS: Take the recommended supplements (optional).

3. MEDICATIONS:

	TAKING	SIDE EFFECT
Antihypertensives		
Antidepressants		
Anti-ulcer drugs		

	TAKING	SIDE EFFECT
Cold/Allergy medications		
Hormones		
Prosexual drugs		
Other		

4. SENSUAL STIMULATION: It's been awhile since you've treated yourself to a massage. Exchange back rubs with your partner this evening. Burn candles, turn the lights down low, put on your favorite music, and shut off the noise of the world. Get out your favorite bottle of scented oil. Devote all your attention to each other's bodies for five to fifteen minutes.

5. EXERCISE: Did you remember to schedule an adventuresome new physical activity for Sunday? If not, do it now. Take the day off from exercise if you like.

Activity: ____

Length of time: ______________________________________

6. SLEEP: If you are still having trouble falling asleep, consider a natural remedy. Enjoy a cup of chamomile tea or Kava Kava Cocoa, take a relaxing bath, or spend a few minutes listening to music at bedtime.

Time to bed: ______ Time awake: ______ Energy level: ______

7. STRESS REDUCTION: Are you becoming more adept and familiar with meditation or yoga? Are you feeling more calm and centered during stressful times? You're only just beginning, so you may not have noticed a difference yet, but yoga and meditation are both excellent methods for taking control of stress. Practice yoga or meditation for at least thirty minutes today. Then describe how you feel:

____

____

____

____

Schedule date night for Saturday.

Book a spa treatment (massage, aromatherapy, facial, or all three if you prefer!) for you and your partner for Sunday.

DAY 27

Thursday

1. DIET: Stay motivated! You're really doing well!

	MEAL PLAN	WHAT I ATE / NOTES
Breakfast	Pineapple-Peach Smoothie* or Fruit Plate	
Lunch	Tabbouleh* Grilled Chicken, Tuna, or Tofu Sandwich	
Dinner	Vegetarian Chili* Steamed Fresh Broccoli	
Dessert/ Snack	Cheesecake Mousse with Raspberry Sauce*	

2. SUPPLEMENTS: Have you been taking the recommended supplements? If so, you ought to be noticing a difference by now. Write about any changes you've experienced below. If you haven't begun, it's not too late to start!

____

____

____

____

3. MEDICATIONS:

	TAKING	SIDE EFFECT
Antihypertensives		
Antidepressants		
Anti-ulcer drugs		
Cold/Allergy medications		
Hormones		
Prosexual drugs		
Other		

4. SENSUAL STIMULATION: Enjoy sensual foods as a prelude to sexual activity tonight. Prepare a variety of bite-sized tasty tidbits such as strawberries, grapes, cherries, kiwis, peaches, chocolate, whipped cream, and other foods that your partner really enjoys. Tie a blindfold over your partner's eyes, then feed him or her the foods slowly and sexually. Let your imagination take over from there.

5. EXERCISE: Consider the level of activity you were engaged in at the start of the program. Have you made progress? If so, congratulations! If not, consider changing an element of your physical fitness routine. Do at least thirty minutes of cardiovascular activity today.

Activity: ____

Length of time: ______________________________________

6. SLEEP: Have you been establishing a bedtime ritual? You might wash your face with warm water, read for twenty minutes, or drink a cup of herbal tea every night just before you go to bed. A regular routine often helps people to fall asleep more easily.

Time to bed: ______ Time awake: ______ Energy level: ______

7. STRESS REDUCTION: Take a time-out today just for you. Do one small activity that you really enjoy, such as getting a manicure, visiting your favorite store, or calling up an old friend. As you do this activity, think about how important it is to treat yourself well. You deserve it!

Activity: ____

DAY 28

Friday

1. DIET: Can you believe that it has already been four weeks since you started the program? Do you feel yourself making progress? Are you pleased with what you've accomplished?

	MEAL PLAN	WHAT I ATE / NOTES
Breakfast	Healthy Milkshake* or Quick Oatmeal*	

	MEAL PLAN	WHAT I ATE / NOTES
Lunch	Vegetarian Chili* Fresh Fruit	
Dinner	Pasta with Green Sauce* Whole-Wheat Herb Bread Fresh Green Salad	
Dessert/ Snack	Chocolate Almond Tapioca Pudding*	

2. SUPPLEMENTS: Take the recommended supplements (optional).

3. MEDICATIONS:

	TAKING	SIDE EFFECT
Antihypertensives		
Antidepressants		
Anti-ulcer drugs		
Cold/Allergy medications		
Hormones		
Prosexual drugs		
Other		

4. SENSUAL STIMULATION: Stop by a florist on your way home today. Pick out a bunch of colorful, fragrant, beautiful flowers. Then take them home and place them in a vase or give them to your partner with a sweet little love note. Put the flowers wherever you'll see them most, whether that is the bedroom, living room, or kitchen. Every time you see them, take a moment to stop and appreciate them. Inhale the aroma. Let your senses come to life.

5. EXERCISE: You've been working hard and deserve a day of rest. Take the day off if you like.

Activity: ____

Length of time: ___________________________________

6. SLEEP: Remember to practice your new bedtime ritual again tonight.

Time to bed: ______ Time awake: ______ Energy level: ______

7. STRESS REDUCTION: Make a resolution that you will share one of your problems or concerns with a companion today. Have a chat with your partner, a co-worker, a friend, a family member, or a professional counselor. Really talk about how you're feeling—try not to gloss over the issues. Don't wait. Do it today. You might also want to discuss your success (or lack thereof) with the Sexual Fitness Program with other program participants online.

DAY 29

Saturday: Date Night

1. DIET: Have you made changes to your eating patterns based on the program? If you have, these changes should by now have formed into habits that you can keep up on your own. Continue the good work and you'll lead a longer, healthier, and more sexually satisfying life!

	MEAL PLAN	WHAT I ATE / NOTES
Breakfast	Ginger Mango Shake* or Whole-Wheat Toast	
Lunch	Garden Fresh Pasta* Green Salad	
Dinner	Crab Enchiladas* Curried Greens*	
Dessert/ Snack	Sensuous Strawberry and Peach Kabobs*	

2. SUPPLEMENTS: Take the recommended supplements (optional).

3. MEDICATIONS:

	TAKING	SIDE EFFECT
Antihypertensives		
Antidepressants		
Anti-ulcer drugs		
Cold/Allergy medications		
Hormones		
Prosexual drugs		
Other		

Even after you've completed the program, you should continue to minimize nicotine, caffeine, and alcohol. You may want to consider keeping up the food and substances diaries on a regular basis.

4. SENSUAL STIMULATION: In preparation for tonight's big date, buy yourself a new outfit. It might be a beautiful new dress or a handsome shirt or even a piece of lingerie or underwear. What it is doesn't matter, as long as it makes you feel sexy. When you put it on, use it to remind yourself that you are a sensual being, desirable and desiring!

5. EXERCISE: Try doing two types of activity for your workout today. For example, do aerobics and lift weights. Golf and do some gardening. Play tennis and go for a brisk walk. You don't necessarily have to exercise for twice as long, but doing two different things should help to keep your energy levels high throughout both workouts. Do at least forty minutes of cardiovascular activity. Challenge yourself.

Activity: ______________________________

Length of time: ______________________________

6. SLEEP: Sleep in for an extra half-hour tomorrow morning if you want.

Time to bed: ______ Time awake: ______ Energy level: ______

7. STRESS REDUCTION: Once again, it's date night. But this one is extra special because it is almost the final day of the program. You've been working hard and making real efforts to improve your sexual fitness, so you deserve a mini-vacation. If you have children, hire a babysitter. You might even consider checking into a hotel or visiting a spa in your area. It doesn't have to be fancy—the point is simply for you to get away from your usual environment. "Home" can be stressful in and of itself simply because the phone rings, people stop by, you can't resist cleaning up, you're tempted by work, and so on. At a hotel or spa, you can get away from these distractions and put all your attention into being with each other. Remember not to have expectations about sexual activity. Simply relax, enjoy the romance, and see where the evening takes you.

DAY 30

Sunday: Celebration Day!

1. DIET: Congratulations! You've completed the Sexual Fitness 30-Day Program. You should be well on your way to enhanced sexual interest, passion, and performance, as well as better health. Celebrate with this delicious and sexually stimulating Aphrodisiac Delight feast or enjoy a meal out.

	MEAL PLAN	WHAT I ATE / NOTES
Breakfast	Mixed Fruit Smoothie* or Whole-Grain Cereal	
Lunch	Noodle Salad with Toasted Sesame Dressing* Fertility Booster Fruit Salad*	
Dinner	***Aphrodisiac Delight!*** Seafood Feast* Easy Asparagus* Whole-Wheat French Bread	
Dessert/ Snack	Apricot Fruit Chutney and Vanilla Nut Whip*	

2. SUPPLEMENTS: Take the recommended supplements (optional). Continue taking them on an ongoing basis with regular supervision by your physician for optimum sexual and general health.

3. MEDICATIONS:

	TAKING	SIDE EFFECT
Antihypertensives		
Antidepressants		
Anti-ulcer drugs		
Cold/Allergy medications		
Hormones		
Prosexual drugs		
Other		

4. SENSUAL STIMULATION: Treat yourself and your partner to a professional spa service today, such as a massage, facial, or aromatherapy. Take the time to relax before and after the treatment. During the service, luxuriate in the sensuality of your own body. Aren't you lucky to have a body that offers you such pleasure?

5. EXERCISE: Today is the day for your big new exercise adventure! You should have set up an appointment with a professional or rented the equipment necessary to try a new physical activity like roller skating, white-water rafting, skateboarding, snowboarding, salsa dancing, bowling, or racquetball. Now's your chance to finally try what you've always longed to do. Do it with gusto. Give it your all. You may discover a new passion or you may just make a fool of yourself—it doesn't matter. What does matter is that you have a good time. It's important to keep challenging yourself. Set the goal of trying a new physical activity at least once a month.

Activity: ____

Length of time: ____

6. SLEEP: Get a good night's rest tonight. You need to keep up your healthy habits from this day forward!

Time to bed: ______ Time awake: ______ Energy level: ______

7. STRESS REDUCTION: You've already got a lot going on today with your aphrodisiac meal, new exercise challenge, and spa treatment. So instead of engaging in any specific stress-reduction activity today, just take a moment to think about how you're doing. Have you learned some effective new stress-management techniques? Do you feel more in control of your life? Write your answers down here, then compare them with what you said on Day 1 of the program. Pick out the most effective strategies for you and pledge to continue practicing them on an ongoing basis.

____

____

____

____

EXTRA: Fill out the Sexual Fitness Survey provided in the *Introduction*. Compare your answers to the ones you gave at the start of the program. Have you improved? Do you feel better about yourself? Are you on your way to Sexual Fitness?

Also, feel free to visit our Web site at www.sexualfitnessMD.com. Let us know how you did. Give us your feedback on your favorite activities. Send us a new recipe. Compare results with others who have completed the program. We'd love to hear from you!

Congratulations! You've done it!

The 30-Day Sexual Fitness Program is just the beginning of a lifelong journey toward physical, mental, and sexual fitness. It is important to maintain the habits you've adopted in the past month on an ongoing basis in order to better your general health and reach your full sexual potential. For many of you, dramatic life changes may have occurred over the last thirty days. For others, you may have started to notice a real difference but will see even greater changes take place in the future. Either way, you will benefit by making these habits a part of your daily life from now on.

You have the power to make the most of your sexual passion, pleasure, and health. Sexual fitness depends on you and you alone. You've done a great job so far, and can continue to do so in the future. Remember, too, that what's good for your sexual health is good for your overall wellness. Let the Sexual Fitness Program be your guide in helping you lead a more healthy and vibrant life.

Keep up the good work!

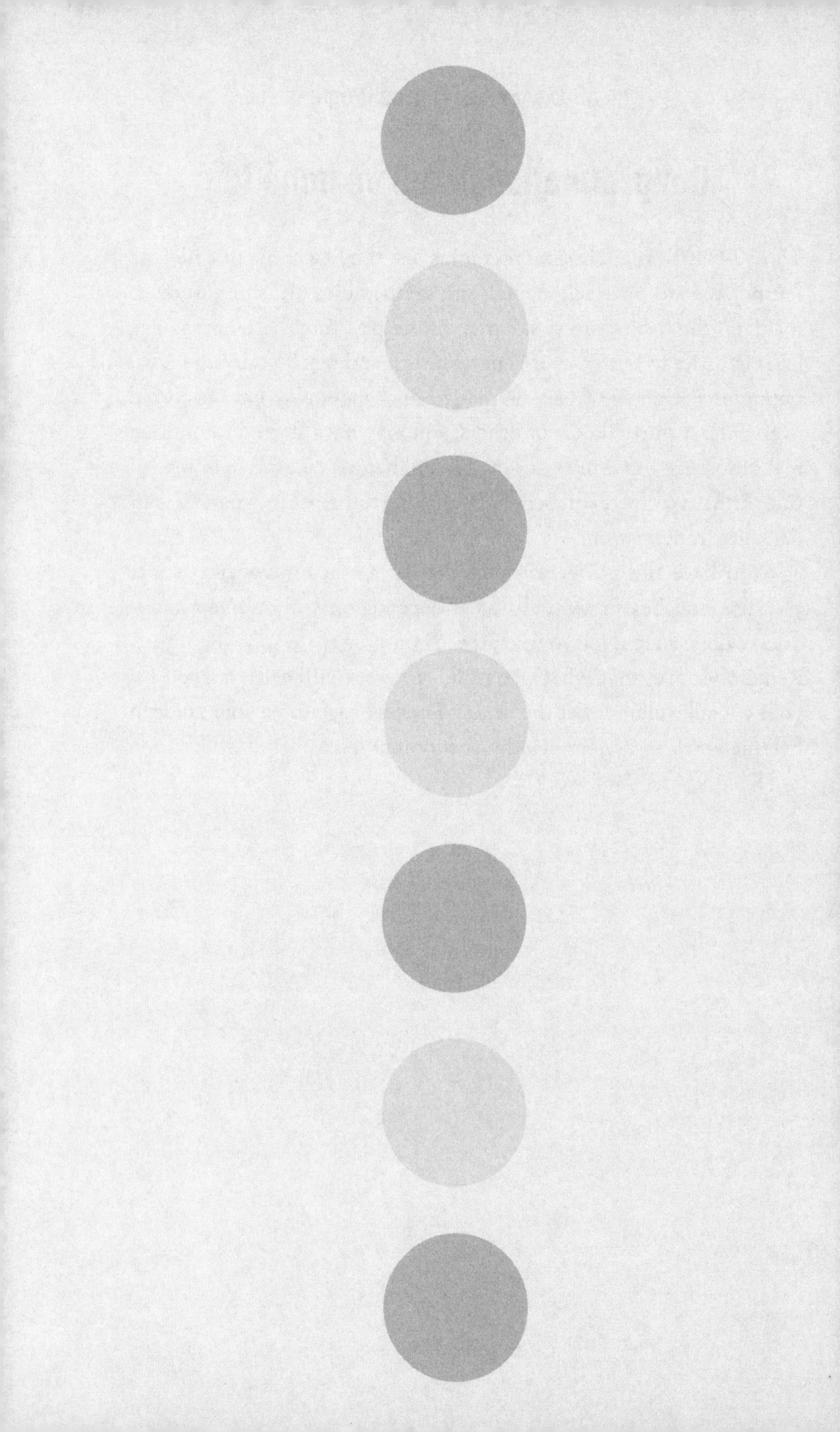

Recipes

Note: In order to make it easier for you to shift the order of recipes or repeat your favorites, we've categorized them by Breakfast, Lunch, Dinner, and Dessert. Recipes are listed in alphabetical order within each category.

Breakfast Foods

Banana Latte

Serves 1

1 cup fat-free milk or soymilk
¾ cup brewed coffee or espresso, chilled to room temperature
1 banana, frozen
6 to 8 ice cubes
¼ teaspoon ground cinnamon

Combine all ingredients in blender and blend until smooth. Serve immediately.

Blueberry Smoothie

Serves 1

1 cup blueberry fat-free yogurt
1 cup fat-free milk or soymilk
1 tablespoon maple syrup
½ teaspoon ground cinnamon
2 cups frozen blueberries

Combine all ingredients in blender and blend until smooth. Serve immediately.

Ginger Mango Shake

Serves 1

¾ cup fat-free milk or soymilk
½ cup vanilla fat-free yogurt
2½ cups diced frozen mango
1 tablespoon fresh lime juice
½ teaspoon ground ginger
1 teaspoon grated fresh ginger
3 to 5 ice cubes

Combine all ingredients in blender and blend until smooth. Serve immediately.

Healthy Milkshake

Serves 1

3 ounces soft tofu
¼ cup toasted wheat germ
1 cup malt or chocolate flavor Ovaltine

1½ cups fat-free milk or soymilk
6 to 7 ice cubes

Drain the tofu and place in blender with remaining ingredients. Blend until smooth. Serve immediately. Use malt Ovaltine for a vanilla shake, chocolate or chocolate-malt Ovaltine for a chocolate shake.

Mixed Fruit Smoothie

Serves 1

1½ cups orange juice
½ cup vanilla fat-free yogurt
1 cup frozen strawberries or other berries
1 banana, frozen
5 mint sprigs

Combine all ingredients in blender and blend until smooth. Serve immediately.

Pineapple-Peach Smoothie

Serves 1

¾ cup peach sorbet
¾ cup white grape juice
3 ounces soft tofu
1 tablespoon fresh lime juice
1½ cups frozen, diced peaches
1 cup frozen, diced pineapple

Combine all ingredients in blender and blend until smooth. Serve immediately.

Quick Oatmeal

Serves 1

½ cup quick oats
1 cup water
Dash of salt
Optional: 1 banana, 8 diced strawberries, or ¼ cup raisins

Combine all of the ingredients in a microwave-safe bowl. Bananas, strawberries, or raisins can be added for extra flavor and natural sweetness. Microwave on high for approximately 2 minutes. Serve with fat-free milk if desired.

Very Berry Smoothie

Serves 1

1½ cups plain fat-free yogurt
2 tablespoons raw honey
1 banana
2½ cups frozen blueberry, strawberry, and raspberry mixture

Combine all ingredients in blender and blend until smooth. Serve immediately.

Lunch Dishes

Asian Cabbage Salad

Serves 2

SALAD:
¼ head green cabbage

¼ head red cabbage
1 tablespoon salt
1 medium carrot, shredded

DRESSING:
2 tablespoons unseasoned rice vinegar
1 tablespoon brown sugar
1 teaspoon toasted sesame oil
1 scallion, minced
2 tablespoons toasted sesame seeds

Shred cabbage. Place in large bowl and sprinkle with salt. Let stand for 1 hour to soften. Drain off excess liquid and wash well in cold water to remove salt. Add shredded carrot. To make dressing, whisk all ingredients together in a small bowl until sugar dissolves. Cover salad with dressing. Let stand for at least 1 hour before serving. Sprinkle with scallions and sesame seeds for final touch.

Asian Green Bean Salad

Serves 2

SALAD:
1 pound fresh green beans
1 tablespoon finely chopped fresh ginger

DRESSING:
2 teaspoons dry mustard powder
1 tablespoon cold water
2 teaspoons sugar
2 tablespoons soy sauce
3 tabelspoons unseasoned rice vinegar
1 teaspoon toasted sesame oil

Trim ends off beans. Boil approximately 5 minutes, until tender but still crunchy. Then drain and chill in cold water. Drain off water and toss with ginger. In separate bowl, combine all ingredients for dressing. Mix well. Toss beans with dressing and serve.

Chinese Chicken Salad

Serves 2

SALAD:

1 head Napa cabbage, chopped
1 romaine lettuce heart, chopped
1 tangerine, peeled and diced, or 1 (16-oz.) can Mandarin oranges, drained
½ cup sliced almonds
½ cup shredded carrots
1 chicken breast, grilled and diced, or 6 ounces firm tofu, drained and diced

SWEET AND SOUR DRESSING:

1 cup unseasoned rice vinegar
2 tablespoons sugar
Dash of toasted sesame oil
Crushed garlic and fresh ginger to taste

Combine chopped cabbage, romaine lettuce, tangerine, almonds, and shredded carrots in large bowl. To make dressing, whisk all ingredients together in a small bowl until sugar dissolves. Add dressing to salad and toss. Top with chicken breast.

Fabulous Fresh Gazpacho

Serves 4 to 6. Use leftovers for other meals if desired.

4 large ripe tomatoes, coarsely chopped
½ yellow onion, chopped
4 cloves garlic, peeled
1 small bunch celery, chopped (hearts only)
1 bunch scallions, trimmed
1 red pepper, chopped
1 bunch cilantro, stems removed
2 tablespoons balsamic vinegar
2 tablespoons olive oil
1 teaspoon dill weed
Dash of sea or kosher salt
Dash of Tabasco sauce
1 ripe avocado, chopped and doused with lemon juice
1 cucumber, chopped
Plain fat-free yogurt

Puree tomatoes, onion, garlic, celery, scallions, red pepper, and cilantro in a blender or food processor. Add vinegar, olive oil, and dill. Season with salt and Tabasco sauce to taste. Blend well. In a separate bowl, combine avocado and cucumber. Pour contents of blender into bowl. Chill. Serve with dollop of yogurt.

Fennel Salad with Herbal Dressing

Serves 2

SALAD:
1 small fennel bulb, sliced
1 small cucumber, sliced
4 scallions, chopped

1 cup shredded carrots
½ pound mixed salad greens or shredded spinach

DRESSING:
1 ripe avocado, peeled and chopped
¼ cup fat-free milk
1 tablespoon fresh lemon juice
1 clove garlic, minced
1 sprig fresh mint
2 leaves fresh basil, chopped, or 1 tablespoon dried basil
Salt and pepper to taste

Puree all dressing ingredients in a blender or food processor. Chill. Combine all salad ingredients in a bowl. Pour dressing over salad and toss. Serve immediately.

Fertility Booster Fruit Salad

Serves 2

4 ounces fresh or canned pineapple, diced
1 kiwi fruit, peeled and sliced
1 apple, cored and diced
1 cup sliced strawberries
½ cup orange juice
1 banana, sliced
2 tablespoons crystallized ginger, chopped
8 ounces vanilla fat-free yogurt

Toss all the fruits and juice together. Top with chopped ginger. Serve with yogurt on the side.

Great Green Quiche

Makes 1 quiche (serves 4 to 6). Use leftovers for other meals if desired.

1 frozen (9-inch) piecrust
1 medium onion, chopped
1 teaspoon olive oil
2½ cups dandelion greens, spinach, or chard, chopped
1 cup grated Swiss cheese
2 eggs
¼ cup fat-free cottage cheese
Salt and pepper to taste
1 teaspoon cayenne pepper

Preheat oven to 350°F. Thaw piecrust and place in pie dish. Bake 5 minutes, then remove from oven. Sauté onion in olive oil. Scoop into piecrust and spread out evenly. Add layer of greens, then layer of grated cheese. In blender, thoroughly mix eggs, cottage cheese, salt and pepper. Pour over greens in piecrust. Sprinkle lightly with cayenne pepper for color and spice. Bake for 35 minutes, until a knife inserted off-center comes out clean and quiche is golden brown.

Health Nut Burgers

Serves 2

Note: If you're in a hurry, simply purchase pre-made veggie burgers.

¾ cup raw, unsalted sunflower seeds
¾ cup walnuts
1 teaspoon ground cumin
1 teaspoon dried oregano

⅛ teaspoon cayenne pepper
2 cloves garlic, minced
1 cup cooked brown rice
2 tablespoons tomato sauce
1 teaspoon olive oil
2 whole-grain hamburger buns

Grind seeds and walnuts into fine meal in blender or food processor. Pour into bowl. Add cumin, oregano, cayenne, and garlic. Mix well. Add brown rice and tomato sauce gradually. Form into 2 patties. Refrigerate for 1 to 2 hours. Brown patties in a skillet lightly coated in olive oil. Serve on buns with lettuce, tomatoes, onions, or whatever fixings you prefer.

Herbed Chicken, Potato, & Olive Salad

Serves 4 to 6. Use leftovers for other meals if desired.

4 skinless, boneless chicken breasts
4 cloves garlic, minced
1 teaspoon finely minced jalapeno or habanero chilies (Be careful to cover your hands with gloves or plastic wrap while chopping chiles and wash hands thoroughly afterwards.)
½ teaspoon ground cumin
1 tablespoon olive oil
2 teaspoons fresh lemon juice
¾ pound red potatoes, cooked
½ small red onion, thinly sliced
¼ cup black olives
¼ cup chopped cilantro
1 small cucumber, chopped
¼ cup fresh lemon juice
1 tablespoon olive oil

Salt and pepper to taste
2 heads curly endive, fresh spinach, or watercress

Preheat oven to 400°F. Marinate chicken breasts in garlic, chiles, cumin, 1 tablespoon olive oil, and 2 teaspoons lemon juice for approximately 15 minutes. Bake on lightly oiled baking sheet for about 20 minutes or grill. Cool for 15 minutes, then slice into strips. Set aside. Combine potatoes, onions, olives, cilantro, cucumber, and remaining lemon juice and olive oil in a bowl. Toss greens with chicken and remaining ingredients. Season with salt and pepper.

Miso Soup

Serves 4. Use leftovers for other meals if desired.

3 dried shiitake mushrooms
1½ cups boiling water
1 carrot, sliced into small rounds
4 cups vegetable stock
4 tablespoons miso
6 ounces firm tofu, diced
¼ cup diced scallions

Combine shiitake mushrooms and boiling water in a bowl. Cover and let stand 10 minutes. Meanwhile, place carrot and 3½ cups vegetable stock in soup pot and bring to boil. Simmer over low heat for approximately 10 minutes, until carrot slices are tender but not mushy. Remove shiitake mushrooms from bowl. Dried mushrooms contain sand, which will fall to the bottom of the bowl during soaking. Spoon the remaining liquid out of the bowl in order to leave off the sand, and add this liquid to the soup pot. Slice the shiitakes into strips and add to soup pot. Simmer approximately 5 minutes. In a separate bowl, combine miso and remaining ½ cup vegetable stock. Pour into soup pot. Add diced tofu and scallions and simmer briefly; do not boil. Serve immediately.

Noodle Salad with Toasted Sesame Dressing

Serves 2

SALAD:

4 ounces soba noodles or fine vermicelli
¼ cup chopped cilantro
¼ cup toasted sesame seeds
4 ounces firm tofu, diced
4 broccoli florets, steamed

DRESSING:

1 tablespoon toasted sesame oil
1½ tablespoons soy sauce
1½ tablespoons balsamic vinegar
½ tablespoon maple syrup or brown sugar
½ tablespoon hot pepper oil

Cook soba noodles according to instructions on package. Drain and rinse with cool water. Combine all dressing ingredients in small bowl and blend until sugar is dissolved. Place noodles in a large bowl. Add dressing, cilantro, sesame seeds, tofu, and broccoli. Toss gently.

Ratatouille

Serves 2

1 small eggplant, peeled and sliced
Sea salt or kosher salt
3 tablespoons olive oil

3 cloves garlic, minced
1 onion, chopped
1 zucchini, sliced
1 tablespoon all-purpose flour
1 green pepper, diced
4 leaves fresh basil, diced
2 tomatoes, chopped or 1 (8-oz.) can stewed tomatoes
4 pitted black olives

Sprinkle eggplant slices with salt and set aside. Heat olive oil over medium heat. Sauté garlic and onion until tender. Toss zucchini slices in flour, then add to skillet. Rinse eggplant slices, pat dry, and lightly dust with flour. Add to skillet. Cook over medium heat for 5 minutes. Cover and simmer for 30 minutes. Add green pepper, basil, and tomatoes. Cook uncovered until all vegetables are tender and liquid has evaporated. Serve with olives as garnish. Tastes delicious warm or cold.

Spinach Salad with Tofu Dressing

Serves 2

SALAD:
1 pound fresh spinach

DRESSING:
2 tablespoons olive oil
2 tablespoons soy sauce
2 tablespoons unseasoned rice vinegar
Dash of hot sesame oil
6 ounces soft tofu, diced
2 scallions, sliced
¼ cup toasted sesame seeds

Wash the spinach, trim the ends, and drain. Set aside. In separate bowl, mix olive oil, soy sauce, and rice vinegar. Add a dash of hot sesame oil, to taste. Stir well. Add diced tofu, green onions, and toasted sesame seeds. Pour over spinach and serve. You may also heat the dressing and serve the salad warm.

Spring Salad with Avocado and Shrimp

Serves 2

1 cup tightly packed spinach, or mustard or dandelion greens
1 clove garlic, minced
1 tablespoon olive oil
2 tablespoons fresh lemon juice
1 hard-cooked egg
Salt and pepper to taste
1 small avocado, peeled and sliced
6 large shrimp, peeled and cooked

Combine spinach, garlic, olive oil, and lemon juice in a medium bowl. Let stand for 15 minutes. Peel and grate egg. Add to salad. Mix thoroughly and season to taste with pepper and salt. Place on plate surrounded by sliced avocado and shrimp.

Tabbouleh

Serves 2

½ cup medium-fine bulgur (cracked wheat)
¼ cup olive oil
8 tablespoons fresh lemon juice
4 scallions, finely chopped
2 bunches parsley, chopped
1 bunch mint, finely chopped

2 large tomatoes, finely chopped
1 cucumber, seeded, finely chopped
Salt to taste

Spread bulgur in a dish. Cover with olive oil and lemon juice. Layer all vegetables over bulgur. Sprinkle salt on top. Cover dish loosely and store in refrigerator for at least 24 hours. Toss before serving.

Tofu-Spinach Pizza Rolls

Serves 2

½ cup pizza or pasta sauce
2 large whole-wheat pitas
½ cup shredded low-fat mozzarella cheese
2 cups spinach leaves
4 ounces firm tofu or feta cheese
½ red onion, thinly sliced
2 tablespoons low-fat Italian dressing
2 basil leaves

Preheat oven to 450°F. Spread pizza sauce evenly over pitas. Sprinkle evenly with mozzarella and spinach. Place on baking sheet. Bake 3 to 5 minutes, until soft but not crisp. Keep warm. In a bowl, toss tofu and onion with Italian dressing. Sauté in a skillet over medium heat for 2 minutes. Sprinkle over pitas. Roll up to enclose filling. Garnish each roll with a basil leaf.

Dinner Dishes

Crab Enchiladas

Serves 2

ENCHILADAS:

¼ pound crabmeat
¼ pound shrimp, peeled and cooked
4 corn tortillas
1 pint fresh salsa
2 ounces provolone cheese, shredded

SOUR CREAM SAUCE:

⅓ cup fat-free sour cream
1 small clove garlic, minced
1 tablespoon minced onion
1 tablespoon chopped cilantro
Dash of sugar

Preheat oven to 325°F. Divide shrimp and crabmeat evenly between all 4 tortillas. Arrange meat down the center of the tortillas in a straight line. Top with salsa and sprinkle with ¼ of the cheese. Roll up each tortilla. Place ½ inch apart, seam side down, in a casserole dish. Pour remaining salsa over top. Cover with foil and bake 20 minutes. Make sour cream sauce by mixing all ingredients in a bowl. To serve, place enchiladas on plates and spoon sour cream over top.

Curried Greens

Serves 2

1 pound spinach, collard greens, or kale
2 cloves garlic, minced

2 tablespoons curry powder
1 cup finely chopped tomatoes
1 tablespoon tomato paste
1 tablespoon brown sugar
1 cup finely chopped onion
1 tablespoon olive oil
¼ pound small new potatoes, peeled and cubed
1 cup water
¼ cup finely chopped cilantro

Wash and drain greens. Cut into 1-inch-long strips. Mix garlic, curry powder, tomatoes, tomato paste, and sugar in a bowl. In a skillet, sauté onions in olive oil until brown. Add tomato mixture, stir well, and cook for 3 minutes. Add potatoes and water. Mix well, bring to boil, then reduce heat, cover and cook for 10 minutes. Add greens and cook for 10 minutes more. Garnish with cilantro.

Dijon-Style Tempeh

Serves 4. Use leftovers for other meals if desired.

1 pound tempeh or 4 boneless, skinless chicken breasts
2 tablespoons olive oil
¼ cup Dijon mustard
2 tablespoon honey
¼ cup cider or balsamic vinegar
2 tablespoons fat-free milk or soymilk

All ingredients should be at room temperature. Preheat broiler. Slice each piece of tempeh in half or pound chicken breasts flat, brush with olive oil, and broil for 5 minutes on each side until cooked. Meanwhile, in saucepan, whisk together mustard, honey, and vinegar. Cook over very low heat until hot. Add milk. Stir thoroughly until heated. Spread tempeh on plates and pour sauce over it to serve.

Easy Asparagus

Serves 2

1 bunch asparagus
2 tablespoons fresh lemon juice
Dash of cayenne pepper

Wash asparagus and break off tough ends. Place on a sheet of microwave-safe plastic wrap. Sprinkle with water. Wrap tightly in plastic wrap. Microwave on high for 2 to 3 minutes, until slightly tender but still crunchy. Immediately remove asparagus from plastic wrap. (Be very careful as the steam is piping hot and can burn you.) Sprinkle with lemon juice and cayenne pepper to taste.

Fiery Fish Fillets

Serves 2

2 large fish fillets, such as red snapper, approximately 2 inches thick
Dash of salt
1 tablespoon cumin seeds
4 tablespoons olive oil
4 teaspoons fresh lemon juice
2 garlic cloves, minced
Dash cayenne pepper

Preheat oven to 375°F. Rinse fish fillets and pat dry. Place in a single layer in a well-oiled baking pan. Sprinkle with salt. Toast cumin seeds in a dry skillet for 3 to 4 minutes, then grind. Mix seeds together in a bowl with olive oil, lemon juice, garlic, and cayenne to taste. Pour marinade evenly over fish, cover with foil, and bake for 20 minutes. Fish should be white and beginning to flake when done.

Garden Fresh Pasta

Serves 2

¾ pound pasta, cooked and drained
¼ cup olive oil
½ cup diced tomato
¼ cup chopped red onion
¼ cup chopped green pepper
¼ cup chopped cucumber
¼ cup finely chopped zucchini
1 tablespoon finely chopped basil
Salt and pepper to taste

Place cooked pasta on large platter. Toss with olive oil. Sprinkle all vegetables over the pasta, saving basil for last. Serve with salt and pepper.

Garden Fresh Stew

Serves 2

8 tiny new potatoes
3 large carrots
2 tablespoons butter
1 small onion, chopped
1 stalk celery, chopped
¼ teaspoon celery seed

¼ teaspoon dried sage
¼ teaspoon dried marjoram
½ teaspoon salt
1 vegetable or chicken bouillon cube
1 to 2 cups water
2 small zucchini, sliced
1 (15-oz.) can garbanzo beans, drained

Place potatoes and carrots, whole, in vegetable steamer. Cover and steam for 15 minutes. Cut carrots into 1-inch slices. Cut potatoes into cubes. Set aside. Melt butter in saucepan. Add potatoes, carrots, onion, celery, celery seed, sage, marjoram, salt, bouillon, and water. Bring to boil. Cover and simmer for 5 minutes. Add zucchini and beans. Return to boil, cover, and simmer for 10 minutes, stirring occasionally.

Grilled Salmon

Serves 2

1 cup sake
½ cup soy sauce
1 tablespoon grated fresh ginger
2 cloves garlic, minced
1 tablespoon brown sugar
2 6-ounce salmon fillets
Lemon wedges

Prepare fish marinade by mixing sake, soy sauce, ginger, garlic, and brown sugar in a bowl and stirring until sugar is dissolved. Rinse salmon fillets. Place in dish and douse with marinade. Cover and let sit in refrigerator for 1 to 3 hours. Drain salmon and discard marinade. Grill fish over very hot coals for about 5 minutes, until salmon flakes when probed with a fork. If you don't have an outdoor grill, wrap salmon tightly in foil and broil for approximately 5 minutes or until fish begins to flake. Serve with lemon wedges.

Vegetarian Chili

Serves 8. Use leftovers for other meals if desired.

2 onions, chopped
1 tablespoon olive oil
3 cloves garlic, minced
2 (15-oz.) cans kidney, garbanzo, pinto, or black beans, or a mixture
1 (15-oz.) can stewed tomatoes
1 cup pasta sauce
3 tablespoons aromatic bitters (can be purchased at a liquor store)
1 tablespoon Worcestershire sauce
1 teaspoon chili powder, to taste
1 teaspoon ground cumin
1 teaspoon dried thyme
1 teaspoon dried oregano
1 teaspoon dried basil
Dash cayenne pepper
2 bay leaves
1 can beer (Note: most of the alcohol cooks off; this is purely for liquid and flavor.)
4 scallions, chopped
1 small bunch cilantro, chopped
½ cup plain, fat-free yogurt

In a large pot, sauté onions in olive oil. Add garlic and sauté lightly. Add beans with the juice, stewed tomatoes, pasta sauce, aromatic bitters, Worcestershire sauce, and all of the spices. Add beer and stir well. Simmer, covered, for at least 3 hours, until liquid is reduced. Chili is best if stored overnight, permitting flavors to develop fully. Serve with scallions, cilantro, and yogurt as desired.

Indian Chicken Curry

Serves 4. Use leftovers for other meals if desired.

1 medium eggplant, cubed
1 onion, diced
1 clove garlic, minced
1 cup chicken or vegetable broth
16 ounces chicken or firm tofu, cubed
1 (15-oz.) can whole tomatoes, chopped
1 tablespoon curry powder
1 teaspoon ground black pepper
½ teaspoon ground coriander
¼ cup chopped cilantro

In a large skillet over medium-high heat, cook eggplant, onion, garlic, and ⅓ cup broth for 5 minutes. Add chicken, tomatoes with juice, curry powder, pepper, coriander, and remaining broth. Bring to boil. Reduce heat to medium. Cook for 30 minutes, stirring occasionally. Top with cilantro to serve.

Island Chicken with Pineapple Salsa

Serves 2

1 (4-oz.) can unsweetened, crushed pineapple, drained and juice reserved
¼ cup minced onions
2 tablespoons brown sugar
1 tablespoon fresh lime juice
½ small jalapeno chile, minced
1 tablespoon minced cilantro
½ tablespoon soy sauce
½ tablespoon honey

½ tablespoon minced garlic
Dash of crushed red pepper flakes
2 boneless, skinless chicken breasts
1 tablespoon cornstarch

Mix pineapple with onion, sugar, lime juice, jalapeno, and cilantro. Set aside. Combine pineapple juice, soy sauce, honey, garlic, and red pepper flakes to taste. Add chicken and coat thoroughly. Stir in cornstarch. Cover and marinate for at least 15 minutes in refrigerator. Remove chicken from marinade and place on the broiler. Put remaining marinade in a saucepan. Grill chicken for 5 minutes on each side or until thoroughly cooked. Meanwhile, bring marinade to boil and cook for 5 minutes. To serve, pour marinade over grilled chicken, then top with pineapple mixture.

Mussels with Vermicelli

Serves 2

1½ dozen mussels
½ cup dry white wine
1 clove garlic, minced
1 scallion, chopped
1½ tablespoons olive oil
2 large tomatoes, peeled and chopped
¼ cup finely chopped fresh parsley
¼ teaspoon dried oregano
Freshly ground pepper to taste
½ pound vermicelli, cooked

Clean and soak mussels. Steam in wine until shells open, about 5 minutes. Remove meat from shells, pull off beards, and trim dark meat. Discard any mussels that do not open. Strain remaining broth and reserve. Sauté garlic and onion in olive oil until onion is soft. Add tomatoes, parsley, oregano, and reserved mussel broth. Cook over medium heat for 10 minutes. Season with pepper. Mix with vermicelli and serve.

Nutty Brown Rice and Spinach Casserole

Serves 4. Use leftovers for other meals if desired.

1 pound spinach leaves, washed
1 tablespoon butter
1 tablespoon all-purpose flour
1 cup fat-free milk
¼ cup balsamic vinegar
½ cup grated Parmesan cheese
¼ cup chopped walnuts
Salt to taste
¼ teaspoon ground nutmeg
3 cups cooked brown rice
¼ cup whole-wheat bread crumbs

Preheat oven to 325°F. Place spinach in kettle with about 1 tablespoon water, cover, and steam until wilted. Drain, squeeze out all water, and chop. Melt butter in a saucepan. Stir in flour and gradually add milk. Stir in vinegar. Mixture will curdle temporarily, but then smooth out. Stir over medium heat until mixture thickens. Add in cheese, walnuts, salt, and nutmeg. Mix spinach and rice into sauce and pour into lightly greased casserole dish. Sprinkle with bread crumbs. Bake for 20 minutes until warm.

Pasta with Green Sauce

Serves 2

1 ¼ cups water
2 scallions, chopped
½ cup shredded romaine lettuce
½ cup shredded spinach
¼ avocado, peeled and pitted
1 tablespoon chopped parsley
1 teaspoon chopped mint
1 teaspoon chopped basil
Lime juice to taste
½ pound whole-wheat noodles, cooked

Blend water and scallions in blender or food processor until smooth. Continue blending at low speed, gradually adding lettuce, spinach, avocado, parsley, mint and basil. Season with lime juice. Toss with noodles. Sauce is delicious served hot or cold.

Penne Pasta with Mediterranean Vegetables

Serves 2

1 clove garlic, minced
2 tablespoons balsamic vinegar
½ cup diced onion
1 small eggplant, diced
1 red pepper, diced
1 cup diced tomatoes
2 tablespoons chopped basil
1 tablespoon olive oil
2 tablespoons grated Parmesan cheese
¼ teaspoon salt

¼ teaspoon dried thyme
4 ounces penne, cooked

Over medium-high heat, boil garlic in vinegar for 3 minutes. Add onion, eggplant, and red pepper. Cook for 5 minutes. Reduce heat to medium then add tomatoes and basil. Cook for 15 minutes, stirring frequently. Stir in olive oil, Parmesan, salt, and thyme. Simmer for 5 minutes. To serve, stir in cooked pasta in sauce and mix well.

Pizza Primavera

Serves 2

1 (14-inch) ready-made pizza crust
1 cup bottled pizza sauce
1 cup shredded mozarella cheese
2 cups vegetables, washed and chopped, in any combination: broccoli, mushrooms, green or red peppers, olives, onions

Preheat oven to 375°F. Spoon pizza sauce evenly onto pizza crust. Sprinkle evenly with shredded cheese. Add vegetable toppings as desired. Bake 10 to 12 minutes, until cheese is golden brown. Let stand 5 minutes before serving.

Roasted Red Pepper Soup

Serves 2

2 cloves garlic, minced
1 small onion, chopped
1 small russet potato, chopped
1 tablespoon olive oil
2 cups water
2 large red peppers, roasted, or 1 (8-oz.) jar roasted red peppers

Salt and pepper to taste
Fresh lemon juice

Sauté garlic, onion, and potato in olive oil over medium-high heat for 10 minutes, stirring frequently. Add water and cook 30 more minutes, until potato is tender. Add roasted red peppers. Puree in blender or food processor. Place in saucepan and simmer over medium heat for 5 minutes. Season with salt, pepper, and lemon juice to taste.

Savory Wild Rice

Serves 2

1 cup dried mushrooms
2 cups water
1 cup mixed white and wild rice
½ cup fresh orange juice
¼ cup dry sherry
½ cup sliced water chestnuts
2 tablespoons chopped parsley
Salt to taste

In a bowl, soak dried mushrooms in water until soft. Squeeze water out of the mushrooms and slice. Dried mushrooms contain sand, so carefully scoop off excess liquid leaving sand in bottom of bowl and reserve. Wash rice well in cold water. Place in pot with mushroom-soaking liquid plus enough additional water to total 2 cups. Add orange juice, sherry, and water chestnuts. Bring to boil, reduce heat, cover, and simmer for 30 minutes. Add mushrooms and cook until rice is tender and all liquid is absorbed. Add parsley and salt to taste.

Scallop Sauté on Steamed Swiss Chard

Serves 2

1 pound Swiss chard
2 cloves garlic, minced
1 ½ tablespoons all-purpose flour
1 ½ tablespoons cornmeal
½ pound sea scallops, rinsed and patted dry
1 ½ tablespoons olive oil
¼ cup chopped black olives
½ tablespoon drained capers
2 teaspoons fresh lemon juice
Freshly ground black pepper

Rinse chard, trim off stems, and chop coarsely. Toss with half of the garlic. Steam or sauté for 10 minutes, until tender. Set aside. Mix flour and cornmeal in a bag. Add scallops. Close tightly and shake to coat scallops thoroughly. Heat oil in skillet. Sauté scallops over medium-high heat for 2 minutes, or until golden brown. Reduce heat to medium-low. Add remaining chopped garlic, olives, and capers. Cook for 1 minute. Spoon over Swiss chard to serve. Season with lemon juice and pepper to taste.

Scalloped Oysters

Serves 2

1 tablespoon butter
1 slice bread, dried and cubed, or ¾ cup ready-made bread stuffing
8 oysters, freshly opened, drained and juice reserved
Salt and white pepper to taste
½ teaspoon finely chopped thyme
¼ cup whole milk

Preheat oven to 375°F. Grease baking dish with butter. Place half of the bread cubes in dish. Add oysters to dish, then season with salt, pepper, and thyme. Cover with remaining bread cubes. Dot with butter. Combine oyster juice and milk. Pour mixture over casserole. Bake 20 to 30 minutes, until bread begins to brown.

Seafood Feast

Serves 2

1 small onion, chopped
3 cloves garlic, minced
3 tablespoons olive oil
½ green pepper, diced
1 stalk celery, finely chopped
¼ cup minced parsley
1 tomato, chopped
⅓ cup tomato paste
1 cup water
2½ cups red wine
½ teaspoon oregano
¼ teaspoon thyme
1 bay leaf
¾ teaspoon salt
¼ teaspoon pepper
8 steamer clams
6 large raw shrimp
4 ounces crabmeat

In large kettle, sauté onion and garlic in olive oil until tender. Add green pepper, celery, parsley, tomato, tomato paste, water, wine, all herbs, salt, and pepper. Cover and simmer 45 minutes or until celery is soft. While soup is cooking, scrub clams, remove shrimp from shells and de-vein. Bring soup to boil. Add crab and clams to pot and cover, return sauce to boil, then simmer for 5 minutes. Add shrimp and simmer for 5 minutes more or until clams open and shrimp turn pink. Serve in large soup bowls.

Shrimp Skillet with Orzo

Serves 2

½ cup onion, minced
1 clove garlic, minced
½ teaspoon olive oil
4 ounces raw shrimp, peeled, de-veined and halved lengthwise
2 tablespoons fresh lemon juice
½ cup white wine
¼ teaspoon salt
¼ teaspoon red pepper flakes
¼ teaspoon dried dill
¾ cup orzo, cooked
2 tablespoons minced parsely
2 tablespoons grated Parmesan cheese

Sauté onion and garlic in olive oil over medium heat. Cook for 5 minutes. Add shrimp and cook for 3 minutes, stirring frequently. Add lemon juice, wine, salt, pepper flakes, and dill. Bring to boil and cook for 2 to 3 minutes. Serve by thoroughly tossing shrimp mixture with orzo, parsley, and Parmesan in large bowl.

Sizzling Tandoori Shrimp

Serves 2

¼ cup peanut oil
¼ cup fresh lemon juice
1 tablespoon grated onion

1 clove garlic, minced
1 teaspoon minced fresh ginger
½ teaspoon ground coriander
¼ teaspoon ground cumin
¼ teaspoon sugar
¼ teaspoon curry powder
Pinch of ground cloves and cinnamon
Dash of pepper
1 small hot red chile, seeded
12 raw large shrimp, peeled and de-veined, or 2 boneless, skinless chicken breasts, cut into 1-inch strips

Puree all ingredients with the exception of the shrimp in blender or food processor. Pour marinade over shrimp and mix well. Cover and refrigerate 3 to 4 hours. Prepare grill with medium-hot coals. Remove shrimp from marinade and place 6 each on metal skewers. Grill approximately 10 minutes, turning and basting with remaining marinade frequently.

Soybean-Vegetable Minestrone

Serves 2

1 tablespoon olive oil
1 small onion, chopped
1 celery stalk, chopped
1 small leek, chopped
2 cloves garlic, minced
2 small Roma tomatoes, chopped
4 cups vegetable stock
2 tablespoons chopped oregano
1 (14-oz.) can cooked soybeans or kidney beans
¼ pound new potatoes, diced

4 ounces shell pasta
3 fresh basil leaves, shredded
1 teaspoon dried parsley
Salt and pepper to taste
Red pepper flakes to taste

Heat olive oil in skillet over medium heat. Sauté onion, celery, and leek in oil for 5 minutes. Add garlic and sauté for 30 seconds. Add tomatoes, vegetable stock, oregano, soybeans, and potatoes, and simmer for 15 minutes. Add pasta, basil, parsley, salt, pepper, and red pepper flakes. Cook for 20 minutes more.

Spinach and Mushroom Manicotti

Serves 2

1 (10-oz.) package frozen chopped spinach, thawed
1 small onion, chopped
1 teaspoon minced garlic
½ cup sliced mushrooms
1 tablespoon olive oil
8 ounces firm tofu or low-fat ricotta cheese
1 tablespoon fresh lemon juice
½ teaspoon salt
¼ teaspoon pepper
1 cup bottled tomato pasta sauce
4 manicotti tubes, cooked
½ cup grated Parmesan cheese
¼ cup chopped parsley

Preheat oven to 350°F. Drain spinach and squeeze out all water. Set aside. In large skillet, sauté onion, garlic, and mushrooms in olive oil over medium heat for about 10 minutes, until onion is transparent.

Add spinach and sauté for 1 to 2 minutes. Remove from heat and set aside. In large bowl, combine tofu, lemon juice, salt, and pepper. Mash well with fork. Lightly oil casserole dish. Evenly spread ½ cup pasta sauce onto bottom of dish. Fill manicotti tubes with tofu mixture and place side by side in casserole dish. Cover with remaining pasta sauce. Sprinkle with Parmesan cheese. Cover pan loosely with foil. Bake for 20 minutes. Remove foil and bake 10 minutes more. Allow manicotti to cool before serving. Garnish with chopped parsley.

Broccoli-Stuffed Potatoes

Serves 2

2 large baking potatoes
2 stalks broccoli
¼ teaspoon salt
1 tablespoon olive oil
1½ tablespoons fat-free milk or soymilk
1½ tablespoons grated Parmesan cheese

Preheat oven to 400°F. Scrub potatoes and make shallow cuts around their middles to make them easier to slice in half after baking. Bake for about 1 hour, until soft. In a hurry? Puncture potatoes, and microwave on high for 15 minutes, rotating once. While potatoes are baking, cut stems off broccoli and break into florets. Steam until tender but still crunchy. Chop into fine pieces. When potatoes are cooked, cut in half. Scoop insides into a medium bowl. Add salt, olive oil, and milk. Mash into smooth paste. Add cheese and broccoli. Mix well. Scoop the mixture back into the potato shells. Bake in 400°F oven until warm.

Desserts

Apricot Fruit Chutney with Vanilla Nut Whip

Serves 2

CHUTNEY:

¼ cup dried apricots
2 pitted prunes
½ apple, sliced
½ pear, sliced
1 cinnamon stick
Dash of nutmeg
1 cup apple juice

NUT WHIP:

¼ cup raw, unsalted cashews or almonds
1½ tablespoons maple syrup
1 teaspoon pure vanilla
1 teaspoon brandy (optional)
1 tablespoon water
Grated fresh ginger to taste

Place all chutney ingredients in pan. Bring to boil. Lower heat and simmer, covered, for 20 to 30 minutes, until fruit is soft and liquid is absorbed. Remove cinnamon stick. To make nut whip, grind nuts to a fine meal in blender. Add maple syrup, vanilla extract, and brandy. Blend well. With blender running, add water a few drops at a time until mixture has a thick, creamy consistency. To serve, put chutney in bowls and top with a dollop of nut whip, then sprinkle with ginger.

Blackberry Crisp

Serves 2

2 cups blackberries or 2 cups peeled, chopped apples
¼ cup sugar
1 tablespoon cornstarch
1 tablespoon fresh lemon juice
¼ cup rolled oats
¼ cup all-purpose flour
2 tablespoons brown sugar
1 tablespoon toasted, chopped walnuts
3 tablespoons butter
1 teaspoon ground cinnamon (Apple Crisp only)

Preheat oven to 375°F. Lightly grease casserole dish. Combine blueberries, sugar, cornstarch, and lemon juice in a bowl. Spoon into casserole dish. Combine oats, flour, brown sugar, and walnuts (add cinnamon for Apple Crisp) in same bowl. Cut butter into mixture. Sprinkle over berries in casserole dish. Bake 45 minutes, until crisp is light brown and bubbly.

Cheesecake Mousse with Raspberry Sauce

Serves 2

½ cup low-fat ricotta cheese
2 ounces fat-free cream cheese
2 tablespoons sugar
½ teaspoon pure vanilla extract
2 cups raspberries
1 tablespoon brown sugar

Puree ricotta, cream cheese, sugar, vanilla, and 1 cup raspberries in blender or food processor. Transfer to bowl. Rinse out blender. Place remaining berries and brown sugar in blender and pulse to lightly chop berries. Layer cheese mixture and berries into 2 dessert goblets. Cover and refrigerate for at least 1 hour.

Chocolate Almond Tapioca Pudding

Serves 2

½ egg, beaten
½ cup packed brown sugar
2 tablespoons quick-cooking tapioca
1½ cups fat-free milk or soymilk
1 square unsweetened baking chocolate, chopped
½ teaspoon pure almond extract
6 tablespoons toasted, slivered almonds

Combine egg, brown sugar, tapioca, and milk in a saucepan and stir together. Let stand 5 minutes. Add chocolate squares. Cook over medium heat, stirring constantly, until mixture comes to full boil. Remove from heat. Stir in almond extract. Let cool for 20 minutes, then stir. Spoon into 2 dishes and sprinkle with almonds to serve.

Grape Sorbet

Serves 2

1 (8-oz.) bunch red or green grapes

Wash grapes, pat dry, remove from stems, and freeze. Place in martini or champagne glasses to serve and eat like sorbet.

Kava Kava Cocoa

Serves 2

3 cups fat-free milk or soymilk
2 teaspoons kava extract powder
2 tablespoons cocoa mix
1 teaspoon pure vanilla extract
Sugar to taste

Heat milk in a saucepan over medium heat. Add remaining ingredients and stir well. Serve immediately in 2 cocoa mugs.

Peach-Blackberry Stew

Serves 2

2 ripe peaches
¼ cup packed brown sugar
¼ teaspoon ground cinnamon
⅛ teaspoon ground nutmeg
1 cup blackberries
⅛ teaspoon grated lemon zest
1 tablespoon toasted, chopped almonds
1 cup red wine
1 cinnamon stick
5 black peppercorns
1 (1-inch) piece lemon peel

Cut peaches in half and carefully remove pits. In a small bowl, mix half of the brown sugar with the cinnamon and nutmeg. Add blackberries, lemon zest, and almonds. Stir gently. Fill peaches with berry mixture and set aside. Combine wine, remaining brown sugar, cinnamon stick, peppercorns, and lemon peel in a saucepan. Stir over medium heat until blended. Pour wine sauce into a sauté pan. Place peach halves in wine, filled-side up. Cover and cook for 15 to 20 minutes, until peaches are soft. Remove peaches from pan. Remove cinnamon stick, peppercorns, and lemon peel from wine sauce and discard. Increase heat to medium-high and reduce wine sauce down to about ¼ cup. Drizzle wine sauce over stuffed peaches and serve.

Sensuous Strawberry and Peach Kabobs

Serves 2

10 large strawberries
2 peaches, sliced
1 tablespoon olive oil

Thread strawberries and peaches onto skewers. Lightly brush with olive oil. Grill over medium-hot coals or in broiler for 2 to 4 minutes, turning frequently until just hot. Serve immediately.

Strawberry-Rhubarb Cobbler

Serves 2

½ cup sliced fresh strawberries
½ cup chopped fresh rhubarb
2 tablespoons sugar
¼ cup maple syrup
½ teaspoon pure vanilla extract
½ tablespoon cornstarch
2 tablespoons peach nectar
½ (9-inch) ready-made pastry crust

Preheat oven to 350°F. In large bowl, combine strawberries, rhubarb, sugar, maple syrup, vanilla extract, cornstarch, and peach nectar. Let stand for 15 minutes. Scoop mixture into small baking dish. Place pastry crust on top. Bake for 20 minutes, until fruit bubbles and pastry is golden brown.

Appendix

A Quick Introduction to Sexual Function and Dysfunction

How exactly does the Sexual Fitness Program work? First we need to understand the basic physiological processes that make sex happen. Then we'll discuss the typical causes of sexual dysfunction. With this background, you'll be able to understand the mechanisms that *Sexual Fitness* seeks to influence. And the better you comprehend what's going on with your body and how the changes you're making are affecting you, the more of an impact the program will have on your personal sexual fitness.

The Basics of Sex

The brain governs the entire sexual experience. Think of it this way: Your brain holds the key for turning on the sexual engine. The sexual arousal process can't even begin unless you have the right key. There are many specific qualifications in order for this key to work. One, the key must have the right design—the situation must be sexual for you, and what this means varies greatly by individual. Two, it must be able to fit the keyhole—you must be receptive to allowing sexual stimuli and thoughts to enter into your head and not be distracted by insecurities, stress, fears, and so on. Three, the engine must turn over and start when you turn the key—your neurotransmitters, hormones, and cardiovascular system must all work properly to get the sexual processes going. Four, you must have a rewarding driving experience in order to use the key again—the sexual experience must be pleasurable and desirable.

When these prerequisites are met, the brain starts sending messages via neurotransmitters to the rest of your body, telling it to go into "excitatory" rather than "inhibitory" mode. Neurotransmitters in the brain, such as dopamine, stimulate the sexual response, whereas others, such as serotonin, inhibit it. This helps explain why certain emotions (e.g., depression, which is frequently associated with low dopamine levels) and medications that affect neurotransmitter levels can influence sexual functioning. A message is sent down the spinal cord, through the nerves, to the various organs involved, including the heart and the genitals. The natural sexual reflexes then unfold.

Similarly neurotransmitters go to work in the genital region. Those released by the parasympathetic nervous system (PNS), such as nitric oxide, promote swelling of the erectile tissue in the vagina and penis. Neurotransmitters from the sympathetic nervous system (SNS) are involved in ejaculation. Sexual medicines make use of these peripheral neurotransmitters. For example, Viagra works indirectly by increasing the level of nitric oxide in the penis to enhance erections. Performing certain activities, such as exercising and eating specific foods, can boost levels of neurotransmitters involved in sex, whereas other activities, such as smoking, can negatively impact neurotransmitter levels.

In addition to neurotransmitters, hormones also play a crucial role in determining sexual functioning. Testosterone, which is known as the male sex hormone because men have about ten times more of it than do women, drives sexual interest and the biological response to arousal in *both* men and women. Increased levels of testosterone lead to more fantasizing, sexual desire, and sexual activity. Estrogen, the female sex hormone, helps make sex comfortable for women—it is important to vaginal lubrication. Abnormally low levels of these two hormones can lead to loss of libido and reduced sexual pleasure. Low levels can also lead to suboptimal ovulation in women and low sperm production in men, resulting in fertility problems. Many of the activities that you do every day, including exercising, sleeping, and reacting to stressful events, impact your body's production of these key hormones.

Your sexual capacity also depends on your cardiovascular health. In order to achieve optimum erections in men and arousal in women, adequate blood flow must be able to reach the arteries of the genital region. Your genitals act like a pump, with blood flowing in through a fine, flexible hose, which are your arteries. When the hose is clogged, blood flow is slowed and therefore arousal is reduced. On the other hand, when your blood vessels are free of cholesterol and your heart is pumping healthily, you are more likely to experience optimum sexual performance. Cardiovascular health depends on consuming a balanced diet, maintaining a healthy weight, exercising, and reducing stress.

Finally, general health impacts your sexual wellness. Often, we don't think about the fact that the body is a connected, unified entity. If one part of your body isn't working—you have a cold, for instance, and your immune system is busy fighting off the virus—then other parts of your body will be affected as well. You won't be able to run as fast or get as much done during the day. At the same time, you won't have the energy or stamina for sex that you do when you're in good physical condition.

Some Causes of Sexual Dysfunction

Many of us are dissatisfied with our sex lives. If you have sexual concerns or simply want to improve your sex life, you are not alone. Typical sexual complaints include low libido for men and women, erectile difficulties and premature ejaculation for men, and vaginal dryness, pain during intercourse and difficulty reaching orgasm for women. And although the causes of these problems vary widely, here are a few of the most common.

1. Neurotransmitter Imbalance

Neurotransmitters are involved in communicating messages from one part of the body to another. Serotonin is a neurotransmitter that makes us feel happy and well balanced. However, it also happens to interfere with sexual drive and response. Anything that causes our serotonin levels to rise above normal has the potential, therefore, to negatively impact sexual fitness. For example, a common type of antidepressant known as a selective serotonin reuptake inhibitor, or SSRI, (brand names include Zoloft, Prozac, and Paxil) works to increase serotonin levels in the brain. This makes many people suffering from depression feel better, but unfortunately a very common side effect is loss of libido.

Dopamine, on the other hand, is a neurotransmitter that plays a key role in sexual motivation and reward. Activities that serve to boost dopamine levels, such as consuming plenty of folic acid, may therefore actually help to enhance your sex drive. Getting a massage or enjoying a great workout are just two ways to increase endorphins, neurotransmitters that deliver pleasure signals to your body and prime you for sexual activity.

2. Low Hormone Levels

As our bodies age, a series of biological, genetic, and lifestyle-related changes occur, all of which can affect our energy levels and overall health. Sex is no exception. As we reach our forties and fifties, our bodies slow down their production of sex hormones, chemicals in our bodies that play a critical role in making sex happen.

Women experience a dramatic drop in hormone levels as a result of reaching menopause, which can have a significant impact on sexual health. Testosterone levels plunge. A lack of testosterone can lead to a lack of desire for sexual activity: Studies show that many women experience a loss of libido during menopause. An 80 to 90 percent decrease in estrogen levels commonly leads to thinning and drying of the vaginal walls, making intercourse painful for some women. In addition, loss of estrogen results in a drop in endorphins, which may make it more difficult for women to enjoy sexual activity. The combined effects of estrogen and testosterone loss can leave many mature women saying, "No thanks, I'm not interested" because sex does not offer enough pleasure for them anymore.

The loss of testosterone happens more gradually for men, but it can still affect their sexual fitness. Men who are testosterone deficient may demonstrate a lack of interest in sex, low frequency of sexual activity and fantasy, and difficulty ejaculating.

Aside from aging, low hormone levels can result from poor nutrition, lack of exercise, stress, and other factors. In order for you to maintain healthy hormone levels, it's important that you focus on all these aspects of your life.

3. Cardiovascular Disease

Our bodies don't work as well for sex when we're not leading a healthy, active lifestyle. Specifically, poor cardiovascular health can have a direct impact on sexual functioning. Cholesterol, which can quickly accumulate with a high-fat diet and lack of exercise, builds up in the blood vessels, clogging them and inhibiting proper circulation. When blood has trouble flowing through the delicate arteries of the body, it can't reach the sex organs in adequate amounts. For men, poor cardiovascular health leads to a very noticeable sexual problem: erectile dysfunction. More than 50 percent of men over the age of seventy have some trouble getting or maintaining erections.

The Sexual Fitness Program

In order to achieve sexual fitness, you need healthy neurotransmitter and hormone levels and a functioning cardiovascular system that will afford you the optimal potential for all of these sexual processes to work. This is where *Sexual Fitness* fits in—whatever you do to maximize your own physiological well-being can help you with your sex life.

- Balance the levels of key neurotransmitters.
- Stimulate the production of critical sex hormones.
- Improve cardiovascular functioning.
- Enhance overall health and wellness.

The 30-Day Sexual Fitness Program, which includes exercises, activities, and nutritional suggestions, is designed to address these fundamental aspects of sexual functioning.

Notes

Introduction: Sexual Fitness

Page 2. Healthy living habits . . . may help you live up to ten years longer. Stamler J, Stamler R, Neaton JD, Wentworth D, Daviglus ML, Garside D, Dyer AR, Liu K, Greenland P. "Low risk-factor profile and long-term cardiovascular and noncardiovascular mortality and life expectancy: Findings for 5 large cohorts of young adult and middle-aged men and women." *Journal of the American Medical Association*, 1999 Dec 1;282(21):2012–8.

Page 3. Marital satisfaction is correlated with sexual satisfaction. Morokoff PJ, Gillilland R. "Stress, sexual functioning, and marital satisfaction." *Journal of Sex Research*, 1998 Feb;30(1):43–53.

Page 3. Couples who engage in regular sexual activity are happier and look younger than their less sexually active peers. Weeks D, James J. *Secrets of the Super-young: The Scientific Reasons Some People Look Ten Years Younger Than they Really Are—and How You Can, Too.* Berkeley, Calif.: Berkeley Publishing Group, 1999.

Page 6. A surprising number of people experience some form of sexual dysfunction. Laumann EO, Paik A, Rosen RC. "Sexual dysfunction in the United

States: Prevalence and predictors." *Journal of the American Medical Association,* 1999 Nov;281:537–44.

Pages 8–9. Are You Sexually Fit? Survey based on a validated diagnostic tool, the International Index of Erectile Function. Rosen RC, Riley A, Wagner G, Osterloh IH, Kirkpatrick J, Mishra A. "The international index of erectile function (IIEF): A multidimensional scale for assessment of erectile dysfunction." *Urology,* 1997 Jun; 49(6):822–30.

Chapter One: Diet

Page 13. "I begged Emilie to give me an oyster . . ." by Lee V (trans.). *Secrets of Venus: A Lover's Guide to Charms, Potions, and Aphrodisiacs.* Boston: Mt. Ivy Press, 1996.

Pages 23–4. Guidelines for Healthy Eating (chart). Roan S. "A Diet for Every Body." *Los Angeles Times,* 1999 June 28:D6.

Page 24. A low-fat diet . . . can dramatically decrease cholesterol levels and even reverse the effects of arteriosclerosis. Schaefer EJ, et al. "Body weight and low-density lipoprotein cholesterol changes after consumption of a low-fat ad libitum diet." *Journal of the American Medical Association,* 1995;274:1450–55.

Page 26. Erectile dysfunction predicts heart disease; high cholesterol levels double a man's risk of ED. Wei M, Macera CA, Davis DR, Hornung CA, Nankin HR, Blair SN. "Total cholesterol and high density lipoprotein as important predictors of erectile dysfunction." *American Journal of Epidemiology,* 1994 Nov 15; 140(10):930–37.

Page 34. Consuming a diet high in soy and low in animal fat can help reduce cholesterol levels. Anderson JW, Johnstone BM, Cook-Newell ME. "Meta-analysis of the effects of soy protein intake on serum lipids." *New England Journal of Medicine,* 1995 Aug 3; 333(5):276–82.

Page 34. Soy combats symptoms of PMS and menopause. Bingham SA, et al. "Phytoestrogens: Where are we now?" *British Journal of Nutrition,* 1998;79:393–406.

Page 34. Garlic may prevent and even reduce the buildup of fatty plaque in the arteries. Efendy JL, et al. "The effect of the aged garlic extract, 'Kyolic,' on the development of experimental atherosclerosis." *Atherosclerosis,* 1997 Jul;132(1): 37–42.

Page 35. A correlation between low antioxidant levels and infertility in men. Smith R, Vantman D, Ponce J, Escobar J, Lissi E. "Total antioxidant capacity of human seminal plasma." *Human Reproduction,* 1996 Aug;11(8):1655–60.

Page 36. Vitamin E supplementation has been shown to improve fertility in infertile males. Kessopoulou E, et al. "A double-blind randomized placebo crossover controlled trial using the antioxidant vitamin E to treat reactive oxygen species associated male infertility." *Fertility and Sterility,* 1995 Oct;64(4):825–31.

Page 37. Low levels of vitamin B-6 are associated with peripheral vascular disease. Robinson K, Arheart K, Refsum H, Brattstrom L, Boers G, Ueland P, Rubba P, Palma-Reis R, Meleady R, Daly L, Witteman J, Graham WE. "Low circulating folate and vitamin B6 concentrations: Risk factors for stroke, peripheral vascular disease, and coronary artery disease." *Circulation,* 1998 Feb 10;97(5): 437–43.

Page 37. Calcium supplementation resulted in a 50 percent drop in women's . . . symptoms associated with PMS. Thys-Jacobs S, et al. "Calcium carbonate and the premenstrual syndrome: Effects on premenstrual and menstrual symptoms." *American Journal of Obstetrics and Gynecology,* 1998 Aug;179(2): 444–52.

Page 38. When people lack dopamine, their sexual interest and pleasure suffer severely. Melis MR, Argiolas A. "Dopamine and sexual behavior." *Neuroscience and Biobehavioral Reviews,* 1995 Spring;19(1):19–38.

Page 38. Reasonable evidence exists for using L-arginine as a dietary supplement to improve male sexual function. Moody JA, Vernet D, Laidlaw S, Rajfer J, Gonzalez-Cadavid NF. "Effects of long-term oral administration of L-arginine on the rat erectile response." *Journal of Urololgy,* 1997 Sep;158(3):942–47.

Page 39. Participants who took magnesium daily for two months noted significant improvement in symptoms of PMS. "Supplements for PMS." *Harvard Women's Health Watch,* 1999 Mar;6(7).

Page 40. Men . . . who took a selenium supplement for three months had healthier sperm and were more likely to conceive. Scott R, et al. "The effect of oral selenium supplementation on human sperm motility." *British Journal of Urology,* 1998;82:76–80.

Page 40. Selenium deficiency can result in infertility, abortion, or retention of the placenta. Bedwal RS, Bahuguna A. "Zinc, copper and selenium in reproduction." *Experientia,* 1994;50:626–33.

Page 41. Low levels of zinc can cause sexual dysfunction in men and may result in infertility. Adequate levels of zinc are also crucial during pregnancy. Ibid.

Chapter Two: Supplements

Page 51. Fifty percent of male subjects with ED who took 60 mg of ginkgo biloba extract a day regained their erections after six months. Sikora R, et al. "Ginkgo biloba extract in the therapy of erectile dysfunction." *Journal of Urology,* 1989;141:188A.

Notes

Page 53. Ginkgo proved extraordinarily effective for both male and female patients suffering from antidepressant-induced sexual dysfunction. Cohen A, Bartlik B. "Ginkgo biloba for antidepressant-induced sexual dysfunction." *Journal of Sex and Marital Therapy,* 1998; 24:139–43.

Page 53. Ginseng caused improvements in penile girth, libido, and sexual satisfaction. Choi HK, Seong DH, Rha KH. "Clinical efficacy of Korean red ginseng for erectile dysfunction." *International Journal of Impotence Research,* 1995 Sep;7 (3):181–86.

Page 53. Ginseng significantly increased sperm count, testosterone, and other sex hormone levels in male patients with fertility problems. Salvati G, Genovesi G, Marcellini L, Paolini P, De Nuccio I, Pepe M, Re M. "Effects of panax ginseng C.A. Meyer saponins on male fertility." *Panminerva Medica,* 1996 Dec;38(4):249–54.

Page 53. Ginseng may help prevent thinning of the vaginal walls during menopause. Punnonen R, Lukola A. "Oestrogen-like effects of ginseng." *British Medical Journal,* 1980;281:1110.

Page 55. Black cohosh significantly alleviated menopause-induced irritability, anxiety, and depression. Tyler V. "Five herbs that ease menopause." *Prevention,* 1999 Mar;51(3):94.

Page 55. Black cohosh works to enhance vaginal lubrication and diminish hot flashes, headaches, and sleep disturbances. Liske E, Wustenberg P. "Therapy of climacteric complaints with Cimicifuga racemosa: Herbal medicine with clinically proven evidence." *Menopause,* 1998;5:250.

Page 56. Ninety percent of the subjects found chasteberry extract helpful in relieving their sore breasts, bloating, and acne. Tyler V. "Chase PMS with chasteberry?" *Prevention,* 1998 May; 50(5):96.

Page 57. Kava induced changes in brain wave activity which were indicative of a sedative state. Saletu B, et al. "EEG-brain mapping, psychometric and psychophysiological studies on central effects of kavain—a kava plant derivative." *Human Psychopharmacology,* 1989;4:169–90.

Page 57. Kava significantly reduces anxiety and enhances well-being. Lehmann E, et al. "Efficacy of a special kava extract in patients with states of anxiety, tension and excitedness of non-mental origin. A double-blind, placebo-controlled study of 4 weeks treatment." *Phytomedicine,* 1996;III(2):113–19.

Page 58. Drinking 300 milliliters . . . of cranberry juice per day significantly reduced urinary tract bacteria levels in older women. Avorn J, et al. "Reduction of bacteriuria and pyuria after ingestion of cranberry juice." *Journal of the American Medical Association,* 1994; 271:751–54.

Notes

Page 58. Drinking cranberry juice for two months reduced the need for antibiotics. Kuzminski LN. "Cranberry juice and urinary tract infections: Is there a beneficial relationship?" *Nutrition Reviews,* 1996 Nov;54(11):S87–90.

Page 58. Subjects who took 400-mg capsules of cranberry extract every day found that their rate of UTIs declined significantly. Walker E, et al. "Cranberry concentrate: UTI prophylaxis [letter to the editor]." *Journal of Family Practice,* 1997 Aug;45(2):167–68.

Page 59. Saw palmetto worked better than a placebo to reduce urinary frequency and nighttime urination. Wilt TJ, et al. "Saw palmetto extracts for treatment of benign prostatic hyperplasia: A systematic review." *Journal of the American Medical Association,* 1998 Nov 11;280(18):1604–9.

Page 60. Reported an increase in sexual desire and performance after taking an oat and nettle supplement. Watson CM. *Love Potions.* New York: Putman, 1993.

Page 61. Men taking 300 mg per day of green oats extract increased sexual activity by 54 percent. Veilleux Z. "Better sex, naturally." *Men's Health,* 1998 Nov:140–42.

Page 62. Fifty-one percent of male subjects taking . . . muira puama daily reported better erections, and 62 percent claimed a boost in their libidos. Carlson M. "Your man." *Vitamins, Herbs and Health,* 1999 Jul;100.

Page 62. Classifies muira puama as "unapproved" for sexual purposes due to a lack of scientific research. Blumenthal M, Klein J, Hall T (eds.). *The Complete German Commission E Monographs: Therapeutic Guide to Herbal Medicines.* Integrative Medicine Communications, 1998.

Page 62. Dong quai can tone the uterus, regulate hormone control, and stabilize the rhythm of the menstrual cycle. Zhu D. "Dong quai." *American Journal of Chinese Medicine,* 1986; XV(3–4):117–25.

Page 63. Revealed no relief of menopausal symptoms with dong quai. Hirata JD, Swiersz LM, Zeil B, Small R, Ettinger B. "Does dong quai have estrogenic effects in postmenopausal women? A double-blind, placebo-controlled trial." *Fertility and Sterility,* 1997 Dec;68(6):981–86.

Page 63. EPO significantly reduced depression, irritability, breast pain and tenderness, and water retention due to PMS. Horrobin DF. "The role of essential fatty acids and prostaglandins in premenstrual syndrome." *Journal of Reproductive Medicine,* 1983 July; 28(7):465–68.

Page 63. Some clinical trials have found that EPO offers no help for women suffering from PMS and menopause. Chenoy R, et al. "Effect of oral gamolenic acid from evening primrose oil on menopausal flushing." *British Medical Journal,* 1994 Feb;308(6927): 501–3.

Notes

Page 64. The German Commission E classifies damiana as "unapproved" due to this lack of conclusive research. Blumenthal M, Klein J, Hall T (eds.). *The Complete German Commission E Monographs: Therapeutic Guide to Herbal Medicines.* Integrative Medicine Communications, 1998.

Page 65. Found yohimbine superior to placebos in treating mild to moderate, but not severe, ED. Ernst E, Pittler MH. "Yohimbine for erectile dysfunction: A systematic review and meta-analysis of randomized clinical trials." *Journal of Urology,* 1998;159:433–36.

Page 66. Yohimbine had no obvious effect on female sexual desire. Piletz JE, et al. "Plasma MHPG response to yohimbine treatment in women with hypoactive sexual desire." *Journal of Sex and Marital Therapy,* 1998;24:43–54.

Page 69. Over 80 percent reported substantial improvements in ability to maintain an erection during intercourse and overall satisfaction with their sex lives. Ito TY, Kawahara K, Das AK, Strudwick W. "A pilot study on the effects of ArginMax, a natural dietary supplement for enhancement of male sexual function." *Hawaii Medical Journal,* 1998 Dec;57(12):741–74.

Ito TY, Kawahara K, Das A. "A double-blind placebo-controlled study on the effects of Arginmax, a natural dietary supplement for enhancement of male sexual function." Scientific Presentation at the Mid-Atlantic Section Meeting and Western Section Meeting of the American Urological Association, 1999.

Page 70. Over 70 percent of participants reported enhanced sexual desire and greater satisfaction with their overall sex lives. Ito TY, Trant A, Polan ML. "A double-blind, placebo-controlled study on Arginmax for Women, a nutritional supplement for the enhancement of female sexual function." Scientific presentation, "New Perspectives In The Management of Female Sexual Dysfunction." Boston University School of Medicine, 1999 Oct. Scheduled for publication in *Journal of Sex and Marital Therapy,* 2000 Fall/Winter.

Chapter Three: Medications

Page 75. About one in four cases of erectile dysfunction are caused by medications. Wagner G, Saenz de Tejada I. "Update on male erectile dysfunction." *British Medical Journal,* 1998;316:678–82.

Page 76. Reference text by Dr. Theresa Crenshaw and Dr. James Goldberg called *Sexual Pharmacology: Drugs That Affect Sexual Function.* Crenshaw T, Goldberg J. *Sexual Pharmacology.* New York: Norton, 1996.

Page 76. Decades of research prove that [antihypertensive medication] increases the rates of erectile and ejaculatory dysfunction in men and decreases desire in both men and women. Lundberg PO, Biriell C. "Impotence—The drug risk factor." *International Journal of Impotence Research,* 1993;5:237–39.

Notes

Page 77. Antidepressants, including tricyclics monoamine oxidase inhibitors (MAOIs), and selective serotonin reuptake inhibitors (SSRIs), can have a serious impact on libido and sexual pleasure. Smith PJ, Talbert RL. "Sexual dysfunction with antidepressant and antipsychotic agents." *Clinical Pharmacology,* 1986;5: 373–84.

Page 77. Wellbutrin (bupropion) is considered to have little or no effect on sexual function. Korenman S. "New insights into erection dysfunction: A practical approach." *American Journal of Medicine,* 1998 Aug;105(2):135–44.

Page 77. St. John's wort . . . is just as effective as standard antidepressants in treating depression, but with fewer side effects. Linde K, et al. "St. John's wort for depression—an overview and meta-analysis of randomised clinical trials." *British Medical Journal,* 1996;313:253–58.

Page 78–79. Sexual Side Effects of Common Prescription Medications (chart). Crenshaw T, Goldberg J. *Sexual Pharmacology: Drugs That Affect Sexual Function.* New York: Norton, 1996.

Page 81. One-third of menopausal women in the U.S. . . . take hormones. Weinstein S. "New attitudes toward menopause." *FDA Consumer,* 1997 Mar.

Page 82. Estrogen replacement therapy (ERT) effectively reduces these symptoms. Coope J. "Hormonal and non-hormonal interventions for menopausal symptoms." *Maturitas,* 1996;23:159–68.

Page 82. In two European studies, postmenopausal women using an estrogen patch reported improved quality of life and sex life. Crenshaw T, Goldberg J. *Sexual Pharmacology.* New York: Norton, 1996.

Page 83. Estrogen-progesterone therapy may increase the risk of breast cancer more than estrogen treatment alone. Schairer C, et al. "Menopausal estrogen and estrogen-progestin replacement therapy and breast cancer risk." *Journal of the American Medical Association,* 2000 Jan;283:485–91.

Page 84. When they are treated with testosterone, these men rapidly regain their interest in sex and ability to ejaculate. Bancroft J. "Endocrinology of sexual function." *Clinics in Obstetrics and Gynaecology,* 1980 Aug;7(2):253–78.

Page 84. Aging men whose testosterone levels are naturally declining respond similarly well to TRT. Swedloff RS, Wang C. "Androgen deficiency in aging men." *Western Journal of Medicine,* 1993;159(5):579–85.

Page 84. Men with already normal to high testosterone levels will not benefit from TRT. Ansong KS, Punwaney RB. "An assessment of the clinical relevance of serum testosterone level determination in the evaluation of men with low sexual drive." *Journal of Urology,* 1999 Sept;162:719–21.

Notes

Page 86. Menopausal women with low testosterone levels report increased libido and sexual responsiveness when given small doses of testosterone. Plouffe L, Simon JA. "Androgen effects on the central nervous system in the postmenopausal woman." *Seminars in Reproductive Endocrinology,* 1998;16(2):135–43.

Page 86. TRT is also effective for women who have had their ovaries removed. Sherwin BB, et al. "Androgen enhances sexual motivation in females: A prospective, crossover study of sex steroid administration in the surgical menopause." *Psychosomatic Medicine,* 1985 Jul/Aug;47(4):339–51.

Page 86. DHEA supplementation . . . can improve overall sense of well-being, inhibit osteoporosis, and stimulate weight loss. Crenshaw T, Goldberg J. *Sexual Pharmacology.* New York: Norton, 1996.

Page 86. As DHEA levels fall, incidence of ED increases. Feldman HA, Goldstein I, Hatzichristou DG, et al. "Impotence and its medical and psychological correlates: Results of the Massachusetts Male Aging Study." *Journal of Urology,* 1994;151:54–61.

Page 87. By the age of sixty, people have less than one-third as much DHEA in their bodies as they did at age twenty. Reiter WJ, et al. "Dehydroepiandrosterone in the treatment of erectile dysfunction: A prospective, double-blind, randomized, placebo-controlled study." *Urology,* 1999;53:590–95.

Page 87. The prohormone effectively raised testosterone levels, increased sexual interest and frequency of sexual thoughts, and enhanced sexual satisfaction among a group of women with low DHEA levels. Arlt W, et al. "Dehydroepiandrosterone replacement in women with adrenal insufficiency." *New England Journal of Medicine,* 1999 Sep;341(14): 1013–20.

Page 87. Andro treatment did nothing to improve sexual function in a group of women suffering from low libido. Bancroft J, et al. "Androgens and sexual behavior in women using oral contraceptives." *Clinical Endocrinology,* 1980;12:327–40.

Page 94. Male smokers are twice as likely to suffer from ED as are nonsmokers. Mannino DM, et al. "Cigarette smoking: An independent risk factor for impotence?" *American Journal of Epidemiology,* 1994;140:1003–8.

Page 94. Smoking causes impotence by restricting circulation. Juenemann KP, et al. "The effect of cigarette smoking on penile erection." *Journal of Urology,* 1987;138:438–41.

Page 94. Moderate smokers . . . experience 20 percent more frequent abnormal vaginal bleeding than expected, and heavy smokers . . . experience 67 percent more. Mattison DR, Plowchalk DR, Meadows MJ, et al. "The effect of smoking on oogenesis, fertilization, and implantation." *Seminars in Reproductive Endocrinology,* 1989 Nov;7(4):293–97.

Page 95. Alcohol generally enhances *psychological* arousal but inhibits *physiological* arousal. Crowe LC, George WH. "Alcohol and human sexuality: Review and integration." *Psychological Bulletin,* 1989;105(3):374–86.

Page 95. It took men significantly more time to reach orgasm after three to four drinks than when they were sober. Ibid.

Page 96. The time it took women to reach orgasm while masturbating increased each time their blood alcohol levels rose. Malatesta VJ, et al. "Acute alcohol intoxication and female orgasmic response." *Journal of Sex Research,* 1982 Feb;18(1):1–17.

Page 96. Alcoholism causes permanent damage to sexual fitness. Van Thiel DH. "Ethanol: Its adverse effects upon the hypothalamic-pituitary-gonadal axis." *Journal of Laboratory and Clinical Medicine,* 1983;101:21–33.

Page 96. Coffee enhanced their sex lives by providing them with extra energy. Crenshaw T, Goldberg J. *Sexual Pharmacology.* New York: Norton, 1996.

Page 97. The more caffeine women consume, the worse the PMS. Rossignol AM, Bonnlander H. "Caffeine-containing beverages, total fluid consumption, and premenstrual syndrome." *American Journal of Public Health,* 1990 Sept;80(9): 1106–10.

Chapter Four: Sensual Stimulation

Page 99. "Various types of nourishing and savory foods."—Susrata. Ratsch C. *Plants of Love: The History of Aphrodisiacs and a Guide to Their Identification and Use.* Berkeley, Calif.: Ten Speed Press, 1997.

Page 102. Gentle touch [and warm temperatures] cause oxytocin levels to rise. Uvnas-Moberg K. "Oxytocin may mediate the benefits of positive social interaction." *Psychoneuroendocrinology,* 1998 Nov;23(8):829–35.

Page 102. Once subjects were allowed to stimulate themselves, oxytocin levels rose steadily. Carmichael MS, et al. "Plasma oxytocin increases in the human sexual response." *Journal of Clinical Endocrinology and Metabolism,* 1987 Jan; 64(1):27–31.

Page 109. Women rate a man's smell as a crucial factor in selecting a new lover. Herz RS, Cahill ED. "Differential use of sensory information in sexual behavior as a function of gender." *Human Nature,* 1997;8(3):275–86.

Page 109. Men rated smell and visual cues as equally important factors in choosing a new lover. Ibid.

Page 109. The smells, not of perfume, but of pumpkin pie, lavender, and black licorice caused the greatest improvements in penile blood flow among the men. Hirsch A. *Scentsational Sex: The Secret to Using Aroma for Arousal.* Boston: Element, 1998.

Page 109. Women's bodies responded most to a strange and unexpected combination of licorice candy and cucumber, followed by baby powder, lavender, and pumpkin pie. Hirsch A, et al. "The effects of odors on female sexual arousal." *Psychosomatic Medicine,* 1998 Jan/Feb;60(1):95.

Page 113. Only in 1993 did they discover the existence of the vomeronasal organ, or VNO, in adults. Wright K. "The sniff of legend: Human pheromones? Chemical sex attractants? And a sixth sense organ in the nose? What are we, animals?" *Discover,* 1994 Apr;15(4):60–68.

Page 114. Within months the trial women's cycles would synchronize with the menstrual cycles of the women whose sweat they wore. Kluger J. "Following our noses. New evidence suggesting the existence of human pheromones, which communicate through the sense of smell." *Time,* 1998 Mar;151(11):72–74.

Page 114. Women who have sex with men at least once a week have more regular menstrual cycles and higher estrogen levels than do women who are not having sex. Cutler WB, Friedmann E, McCoy NL. "Pheromonal influences on sociosexual behavior in men." *Archives of Sexual Behavior,* 1998 Nov; 27(1):1–12.

Page 117. When the subjects listened to positive mood music . . . they experienced greater penile tumescence and reported that they were more aroused than when not listening to music. Mitchell WB, DiBartolo PM, Brown TA, Barlow DH. "Effects of positive and negative mood on sexual arousal in sexually functioning males." *Archives of Sexual Behavior,* 1998;27(2):197–207.

Page 120. How Colors Influence Sexual Arousal (chart). Watson CM. *Love Potions.* New York: Putnam, 1993.

Chapter Five: Exercise

Page 128. After nine months of regular workouts, these men engaged in more frequent sexual activity, had fewer problems with erectile dysfunction (ED), and reported a higher percentage of satisfying orgasms. White JR, Case DA, McWhirter D, Mattison AM. "Enhanced sexual behavior in exercising men." *Archives of Sexual Behavior,* 1990 Nov 3;19:193–207.

Page 128. Eating a healthy diet and exercising regularly will significantly lower levels of "bad" LDL cholesterol while increasing or maintaining levels of "good" HDL cholesterol. Stefanick ML, et al. "Effects of diet and exercise in men and postmenopausal women with low levels of HDL cholesterol and high levels of LDL cholesterol." *New England Journal of Medicine,* 1998;339:12–20.

Notes

Page 129. Men's testosterone levels increased during exercise, peaking at twenty to thirty minutes after the session and then declining. Cumming DC, Brunsting LA, Strich G, Ries AL, Rebar RW. "Reproductive hormone increases in response to acute exercise in men." *Medicine and Science in Sports and Exercise,* 1986 Aug;18(4):369–73.

Page 129. Women's testosterone levels [were] significantly higher fifteen to thirty minutes after physical activity. Cumming DC, Wall SR, Galbraith MA, Belcastro AN. "Reproductive hormone responses to resistance exercise." *Medicine and Science in Sports and Exercise,* 1987;19(3):234–38.

Page 129. For a majority of women, exercising regularly effectively reduces hot flashes, sweating, and mood swings caused by menopause. Wilbur J, Holm K, Dan, A. "The relationship of energy expenditure to physical and psychologic symptoms in women at midlife." *Nursing Outlook,* 1992 Nov/Dec;40(6):269–76.

Page 131. Self-rated sexual satisfaction and physical fitness were highly correlated, even in the seventy-plus age group. Bortz WM, Wallace DH. "Physical fitness, aging, and sexuality." *Western Journal of Medicine,* 1999;170:167–69.

Page 134. Engaging in moderate-intensity exercise reduces your risk of heart disease just as effectively as high-intensity exercise does. Lemaitre RN, et al. "Leisure-time physical activity and the risk of primary cardiac arrest." *Archives of Internal Medicine,* 1999 Apr;159(7):686–90.

Page 135. The farther the men walked, the more their heart disease risk fell: a 15 percent decrease for every half mile covered. Hakim A, et al. "Effects of walking on coronary heart disease in elderly men: The Honolulu Heart Program." *Circulation,* 1999 July 6;100(1):9–13.

Page 135. Women, walking regularly . . . and at a brisk pace, significantly reduced the incidence of heart disease. Manson JE, et al. "A prospective study of walking as compared with vigorous exercise in the prevention of coronary heart disease in women." *The New England Journal of Medicine,* 1999 Aug 26;341:650–58.

Page 135. Sedentary adults over age sixty [who] did t'ai chi . . . experienced a reduction in blood pressure just as significant as did a group participating in an equal amount of aerobic exercise. Young DR, Appel LJ, Jee SH, Miller ER. "The effects of aerobic exercise and t'ai chi on blood pressure in older people: Results of a randomized trial." *Journal of the American Geriatrics Society,* 1999 Mar;47(3): 277–84.

Page 136. After sixteen weeks, the women in the lifestyle group had lost just as much weight as the aerobic exercise group, and their cholesterol levels were significantly reduced. Andersen RE, et al. "Effects of lifestyle activity vs. structured aerobic exercise in obese women: A randomized trial." *Journal of the American Medical Association,* 1999 Jan 27;281(4):335–40.

Page 136. Those in the lifestyle group demonstrated similar improvements in activity level, cardiorespiratory fitness, and blood pressure to the structured activity group. Dunn AL, et al. "Comparison of lifestyle and structured interventions to increase physical activity and cardiorespiratory fitness: A randomized trial." *Journal of the American Medical Association*, 1999 Jan 27;281(4):327–34.

Page 140–141. Recommended Weight Based on Height Men and Women (charts). Copyright Metropolitan Life Insurance Company.

Page 142. Men and women who are severely underweight typically experience loss of libido and fertility. Frisch RE. "Fatness and fertility." *Scientific American*, 1988 Mar;258(3): 88–95.

Page 142. When people lost enough weight to bring themselves to within ten pounds of their target weight, their level of sexual interest and activity rose substantially. Abramson EE, Catalano S. "Weight loss and sexual behavior." *Journal of Obesity and Weight Regulation*, 1985 Winter;4(4):268–73.

Chapter Six: Sleep

Page 145. "Blessings on him who invented sleep . . ."—Cervantes. Bartlett J, Kaplan J. *Bartlett's Familiar Quotations.* New York: Little, Brown, 1992.

Page 145. Forty-three percent of Americans say they usually sleep only six or fewer hours a night. Kate NT. "To reduce stress, hit the hay." *American Demographics,* 1994 Sept;16(9):14–15.

Page 147. Healthy sleep is the most powerful predictor of longevity. Dement WC, Vaughan C. *The Promise of Sleep.* New York: Simon & Schuster, 1999.

Page 148. The Stanford Sleepiness Scale (chart). Ibid.

Page 149. Sleep Calendar (chart). Developed by The National Sleep Foundation.

Page 151. Healthy men who were deprived of sleep for forty-eight-hour periods experienced a significant drop in testosterone levels. Gonzalez-Santos MR, Gaja-Rodriguez OV, Alonso-Uriarte R, Sojo-Aranda I, Cortes-Gallegos V. "Sleep deprivation and adaptive hormonal responses of healthy men." *Archives of Andrology,* 1989;22(3):203–7.

Page 151. Forty-four percent of people with sleep-disordered breathing . . . suffer from decreased libido and/or erectile dysfunction (ED). Ferguson KA, Fleetham JA. "Sleep-related breathing disorders 4: Consequences of sleep disordered breathing." *Thorax,* 1995 Sept;50(9):998–1004.

Notes

Page 151. Women who worked night shifts took significantly longer to become pregnant. Bisanti L, et al. "Shift work and subfecundity: A European multicenter study." *Journal of Occupational and Environmental Medicine,* 1996 Apr; 38(4):352–58.

Page 151. Many other studies have discovered a correlation between night shift work and unfavorable pregnancy outcomes. Bodin L, Axelsson G, Ahlborg G Jr. "The association of shift work and nitrous oxide exposure in pregnancy with birth weight and gestational age." *Epidemiology,* 1999 Jul;10(4):429–36. Nurminen T. "Shift work, fetal development and course of pregnancy." *Scandanavian Journal of Work, Environment, and Health,* 1989;15:395–403.

Page 151. A study of college students found a strong correlation between high-quality sleep and overall health and sense of well-being. Pilcher JJ, Ott ES. "The relationships between sleep and measures of health and well-being in college students: A repeated measures approach." *Behavioral Medicine,* 1998 Winter;23(4):170–77.

Page 152. Forty-eight percent of Americans say they experience insomnia occasionally, and almost one-quarter claim to suffer from it every night. "Omnibus Sleep in America Poll." National Sleep Foundation, 1998.

Page 153. ERT reduces hot flashes, enhances the quality of sleep, and decreases the frequency of nighttime arousal. Polo-Kantola P, et al. "Effect of short-term transdermal estrogen replacement therapy on sleep: A randomized, double-blind crossover trail in postmenopausal women." *Fertility and Sterility,* 1999 May;71(5):873–80.

Page 153. Both men and women claimed that, more than anything else, the stress and worries of everyday life . . . caused them to lose sleep. Urponen H, Vuori I, Hasan J, Partinen M. "Self-evaluations of factors promoting and disturbing sleep: An epidemiological survey in Finland." *Social Science and Medicine,* 1988;26(4):443–50.

Page 155. Benzodiazepine sedatives, the most commonly prescribed type of sleeping pills, can interfere with sexual desire and response. Crenshaw TL, Goldberg JP. *Sexual Pharmacology.* New York: Norton, 1996.

Page 158. When people slept with neck support pillows they reported more sound quality sleep than when sleeping with regular pillows. Persson L, Moritz U. "Neck support pillows: A comparative study." *Journal of Manipulative and Physiological Therapeutics,* 1998 May;21(4):237–40.

Page 159. Women [who] wore a sun visor . . . demonstrated a significant increase in sleep duration and quality. Cooke KM, Kreydatus MA, Atherton A, Thoman EB. "The effects of evening light exposure on the sleep of elderly women expressing sleep complaints." *Journal of Behavioral Medicine,* 1998 Feb;21(1):103–14.

Page 160. Most people who exercise feel that it has a greater positive impact on sleep than any single other factor, including a good day at work or a quiet sleeping environment. Urponen H, Vuori I, Hasan J, Partinen M. "Self-evaluations of factors promoting and disturbing sleep: An epidemiological survey in Finland." *Social Science and Medicine,* 1988;26(4):443–50.

Page 160. Those who followed an exercise training program slept better and longer than did a control group. King AC, et al. "Moderate-intensity exercise and self-rated quality of sleep in older adults: A randomized controlled trial." *Journal of the American Medical Association,* 1997 Jan 1;277(1):32–37.

Page 161. Smokers tend to have problems going to sleep and staying asleep, and report high levels of daytime sleepiness. Phillips BA, Danner FJ. "Cigarette smoking and sleep disturbance." *Archives of Internal Medicine,* 1995 Apr;155(7):734–37.

Page 162. Warm feet proved more effective in putting a group of men to sleep than did treatment with light or melatonin. Krauchi K, et al. "Warm feet promote the rapid onset of sleep." *Nature,* 1999 Sept 2;401(6748):36–37.

Page 162. Massage helps people sleep better. Griffin K. "Hands-on healing." *Health,* 1995 Oct;9(6):59–63.

Chapter Seven: Stress Reduction

Page 165. Six in ten adults in the United States say they feel under great stress at least once a week. Kate NT. "To reduce stress, hit the hay." *American Demographics,* 1994 Sept;16(9): 14–15.

Page 165. Stress is highly correlated [with sexual dysfunction]. Laumann EO, Paik A, Rosen RC. "Sexual dysfunction in the United States: Prevalence and predictors." *Journal of the American Medical Association,* 1999 Feb 10;281(6):537–44.

Page 165. Humans simply did not evolve to be able to cope with the constant daily stress of our modern lives. Sapolsky R. *Why Zebras Don't Get Ulcers: An Updated Guide to Stress, Stress-Related Diseases, and Coping.* New York: W.H. Freeman & Co, 1998.

Page 169. Cortisol stimulates the body's metabolism, but also suppresses production of testosterone. Rabin D, Gold PW, Margioris AN, Chrousos GP. "Stress and reproduction: Physiologic and pathophysiologic interactions between the stress and reproductive axes." *Mechanisms of Physical and Emotional Stress,* Chrousos GP (ed). New York: Plenum Press, 1988.

Page 169. Sperm concentration and total number of active sperm decreased significantly when self-reported stress increased. Clarke RN, Klock SC, Geoghegan A, Travassos DE. "Relationship between psychological stress and semen quality among in-vitro fertilization patients." *Human Reproduction,* 1999 Mar;14(3):753–58.

Notes

Page 169. Women who work in jobs they consider to be stressful tend to have less-regular menstrual cycles than do women who work in jobs that they consider low-anxiety. Matteo S. "The effect of job stress and job interdependency on menstrual cycle length, regularity, and synchrony." *Psychoneuroendocrinology,* 1987;12 (6):467–76.

Page 169. Working long hours (more than seventy-one hours per week) increased the time in took them to conceive. Tuntiseranee P, Olsen J. "Are long working hours and shift work risk factors for subfecundity? A study among couples from southern Thailand." *Occupational and Environmental Medicine,* 1998 Feb;55(2):99–105.

Page 170. Women who rated themselves as under a great deal of stress were twelve times more likely to miscarry early in their pregnancies than were less stressed women. Hjollund NH, et al. "Distress and reduced fertility: A follow-up study of first-pregnancy planners." *Fertility and Sterility,* 1999;72(1):47–53.

Page 171. The more men and women needed to concentrate on complicated tasks, the less they responded to erotic stimuli. Elliott AE, O'Donohue WT. "The effects of anxiety and distraction on sexual arousal in a nonclinical sample of heterosexual women." *Archives of Sexual Behavior,* 1997;26(6):607–24.

Page 173. Maintaining healthy habits such as these helps reduce symptoms of and improve ability to cope with stress. McEwen BS. "Protective and damaging effects of stress mediators." *New England Journal of Medicine,* 1988;338(3):171–78.

Page 173. People who are aerobically fit have less of a physiological response to and faster recovery from stress than do the unfit. Senkfor AJ, Williams JM. "The moderating effects of aerobic fitness and mental training on stress reactivity." *Journal of Sport Behavior,* 1995 June;18(2):130–57.

Page 175. Social support is one of the most effective methods of reducing stress. Morokoff PJ, Gillilland R. "Stress, sexual functioning, and marital satisfaction." *Journal of Sex Research,* 1998 Feb;30(1):43–53.

Page 176. Pet owners had a higher survival rate one year after hospital discharge than did nonowners. Bower B. "Stress goes to the dogs." *Science News,* 1991 Nov 2;140 (18):285.

Page 181. Meditation has been reported to lower blood pressure and heart rate, improving circulation by causing blood vessels to relax. Barnes V, et al. "Acute effects of transcendental meditation on hemodynamic functioning in middle-aged adults." *Psychosomatic Medicine,* 1999 Jul/Aug;61(4):524–31.

Page 185. Laughter also has a direct impact on stress by reducing muscle tension and blood pressure and lowering levels of stress hormones. Berk LS, Tan SA, Fry WF, Napier BJ, Lee JW, Hubbard RW, Lewis JE, Eby WC. "Neuroendocrine and stress hormone changes during mirthful laughter." A*merican Jounral of Medical Science,* 1989 Dec;298(6):390–96.

Notes

Page 185. When you're being social you're thirty times more likely to laugh. Roach M. "The laughing clubs of India." *Health,* 1996 Sept;10(5):93–96.

Page 186. After twelve weeks [of listening to classical music], all of them reported feeling less fatigue and depression, and were in a better overall mood. "Or you could have a martini." *Forbes,* 1998 May 4;161(9):86.

Page 187. Bathing [in warm water] relieves muscle tension, enhances circulation by dilating blood vessels, and can even improve your mood. Hooper PL. "Hot-tub therapy for Type 2 diabetes mellitus. *New England Journal of Medicine,* 1999 Sept 16;341(12):924–25.

Page 188. Kava has been proven a powerful tool for relieving anxiety. Saletu B, et al. "EEG-brain mapping, psychometric and psychophysiological studies on central effects of kavain—A kava plant derivative." *Human Psychopharmacology,* 1989;4:169–90.

Index

Index

Index

Index

Index

Index

Index